MRS H'S STORM IN A D CUP

JOANNE HINDS

To Karen
Please enjoy my story

Much Love
Joanne Hinds
AKA
"Mrs H"

JOANNE HINDS

Chapter 1 - January 2021
Chapter 2 - Magseed
Chapter 3 - The 'Obligatory' Covid Test
Chapter 4 - Feeling Disappointed
Chapter 5 - The Actual Covid Test
Chapter 6 - Surgery Day & Bra Buying
Chapter 7 - February 2021
Chapter 8 - Two Weeks Post Surgery
Chapter 9 - Meet the Oncologist
Chapter 10 - Let's Get Wiggy With It
Chapter 11 - Feeling Blessed
Chapter 12 - Chemotherapy
Chapter 13 - Scared of Stalybridge but actually Terrified of Tameside
Chapter 14 - Chemo 1 – First Cycle – 7 May 2021
Chapter 15 - Chemo – Cycles 2 & 3
Chapter 16 - Chemo – Cycles 4 & 5 at 'The Mother Ship'
Chapter 17 - Chemo 6 – The last One
Chapter 18 – Radiotherapy
Chapter 19 - Moving On
Chapter 20 - April/May 2022

JOANNE HINDS

FOREWARD

Hello and welcome to my book, 'Mrs H's - Storm in a D Cup' – it's my first ever attempt so you will have to bear with me if I sometimes go off piste slightly. Don't forget, I am not doing an A Level Creative Writing Course, so if you happen upon a spelling mistake or some dodgy grammar, or the tenses trip from one to another, just ignore and crack on. For the teachers in my family, please rid yourself of the urge to get your best red marking pen out!!

I suppose you could say then that it is an 'Autobiography' of my life, but you don't have to worry because I am not going to bore you with the first 57 years. It will just be my 58/59th year. The year when life was upside down and unprecedented, not just for me, but also for all of us.

The VID was still rearing its ugly head and we were still in the midst of a Global Pandemic.

We had had almost 12 months of being in a lockdown situation which hopefully we will never see the likes again.

Mr H was able to work from home as he works for

himself and thankfully, kept busy. He set himself up in one of the bedrooms and I set up camp in the kitchen. We coped well I think. Obviously, like everyone else, not seeing friends and family was tough, but at least we liked being in each other's company which was a bonus, and it didn't have such a massive impact on us.

We did, however, have plenty of opportunity to see people over the 'Zoom' – it was like an episode of Celebrity Squares every week, as we held quizzes every Monday night for about 3 months and then when the 'tiering' (controversial) lessened and people were given that little bit of freedom, we moved them to monthly, right up until Christmas. Looking back, I don't know how we did it. Mr H being the whiz he is, or nerd, as I like to call him prepared the questions and loaded up the computer system. It was all very technical. The questions were multiple choice and you answered them on your phone. Clever.

Whilst he was nerding, I was head of recruitment, admin and finance. As well as having a good time and keeping in touch with friends, we raised £3,251 for Willow Wood.

One of the hardest parts of lockdown was not being able to see family, especially the older ones who were not local to us. Mrs H Snr lives over in Northwich and she was lucky, in that she had Mr H's sister and brother-in-law nearby and my Aunty Jose, who lives over in Knott End on Sea, had lovely young neighbours who looked after her and became quite apt at doing a Morrisons order too.

In the 'real world' as I now like to call it, Aunty Jose who is a sprightly 81, not that you would ever guess, in her words 'looks after the old folk' in the village. I am not actually sure what age you have to be to qualify for that title though. She is now back dog minding, prescription collecting, taxi service to hospitals and lots more. She is also back golfing twice a week, weather permitting. She is a wonder to behold and if I am half the woman she is, I will have done ok. She will kill me for saying this, but she is actually half the woman I am, as she only comes up to just under my shoulder☺

Back to lockdown

I remember right back at the beginning when we heard the first rumblings of this mystery illness. I remember telling Aunty Jean (not a real Aunty but if you knew her, you would wish she was yours which is why I am trying to get her to adopt me) that it was nothing and it would be over before we knew it. Ever the optimist! How wrong was I?

Apologies, dad joke on the way:

Nail salons, hair salons, waxing centres and tanning places are closed.

It's about to get ugly out there ☺

As the days turned into weeks, and the weeks turned into months, those of us who like a trip to the hair salon or beauty shops were beginning to get a bit jittery. That 6 week trim and colour touch up that happened come what may, went straight out the window, unless you had the luxury of living with someone who was trustworthy with the scissors and the supermarket colour (if you could get hold of them). I am sure if we could have got out and seen people in person there would have been some dodgy fringes going on too.

Eyebrows were starting to crawl across faces like slugs, which apparently in some circles is actually 'on trend' and previously manicured nails were a thing we only dreamed of. Not technically true in my case, as I actually have an 'Ology' as I like to call it, in Beauty Therapy & Cosmetology, from back in my youth and childhood, hence the ology☺ so mine were always spot on. It was only a part time evening course but we had all the gear and uniform. A dodgy white therapists dress, white tights and white shoes – classy. My dad used to say that I looked like I was going working in a chippy☺

Back to hair, there are probably many of you that for

years, have been disguising your greying temples in an attempt to find some kind of 'eternal youth'. That regular trip to the salon to make you feel young and glamourous.

Therefore, if you thought I was a natural blonde, well you are sadly mistaken. That grey popped out quicker than a jelly out of a trifle. Lucky for me though, I had Mr (Vidal) Hinds to hand. He put on his apron and rubber gloves and set about me 'locks' like a right professional. I must say, he made a mighty fine job of it. As much as I trust him, I drew the line at letting him attack me with the scissors.

His hair seemed to be sprouting more than usual, or was it just that we were seeing more of each other than we would have normally. No trips to the 'Majestic Barbers' down in the Bridge, as sadly closed for the duration like lots of other establishments.

He decided to invest in a good pair of clippers and worked out that I would only need to use them on him about 3 times to be in profit. Great, he would be saving in the long-run. I was under immense pressure not to make a hash of things. One slip in the wrong direction and that would be it. I suppose I could have blagged that I was trying to give him some kind of 'Nike' stripe (Whoops, product placement alert, not that I am any sort of influencer!) I remembered one particular barber who used to have the privilege of coiffuring Mr H's flowing locks (he wishes), commenting that 'the shape of his head, ruined his haircut'!! What hope did I have? In actual fact, I think I did quite well, under supervision of course, but I don't think I will be any threat to the local barbers.

Just for the record, said hair clippers were ordered via everyone's new best friend – Amazon. In fact, during lockdown at Hindsy Towers, we went from not really purchasing online, to having a delivery almost every day. On one particular day, it got to around 5pm and I said with shock and horror to Mr H that there must be something wrong as we had not had a delivery and that Amazon shares would be dipping.

Back to lockdown a second time!

As I have previously mentioned, in the absence of not having older family locally to look after, we turned into a temporary 'Meals on Wheels' service for some of my wonderful 'mature' friends. I have to call them that or at least one of them will kill me. Every Sunday we set about deciding what meal we would prepare for lunch for ourselves and for them too. In a way it forced us into having a full, all the trimmings Sunday lunch each week. We prepped and cooked, plated up and delivered to my lovely friends Aunty Jean and Arthur and Arthur's friend Peter. Mr H even put on his striped apron and chef's hat, donning a tea towel over his arm. Proper looked the part. We shopped for them when required and I didn't mind standing in those queues at the supermarket. It seems like a dream now, or should I say nightmare, and I can hardly believe that is what we had to do.

So then imagine, when we (my husband and I – whoops I sound quite Regal there) were toddling along doing the best we could to stay safe, neither of us having contracted 'The VID' when *'BOOM',* I was diagnosed with breast cancer in the January of 2021.

When you are given this kind of a diagnosis, or anything that could be life changing, your world momentarily stops. Your usual trustworthy, sensible brain stops computing and you immediately think the worst. It's the end. Your heart pounds and eyes burn. You don't listen properly to what is being said to you and you fall into some kind of parallel world, with plates spinning around your head. I cannot properly describe the feelings that you get in this darkest of moments: numb, distraught, frantic, the list is endless – a fusion of emotions. However, once you calm down and get over the initial shock, and I can only say this from personal experience, things do start to make some kind of sense. Things do get better, or if not better, easier.

During the ensuing months, I posted a few lengthy blogs, or whatever you want to call them to let my wider group of friends know what was happening.

The main reason however, was to highlight the need for women to attend their mammogram appointments, for this indeed was where my blighter was picked up – a routine mammogram, not a lump in sight. How lucky am I, that it was my turn. It was also to reiterate that if you ever have a worry about anything or feel something is not quite right, pick that phone up and get yourself checked. Easier said than done but really important. My mantra therefore is:

'If in doubt, check it out'

Having not really written anything of any real length or substance before, I was quite surprised when many of my friends said that they loved reading my posts and that apparently I had a 'knack for writing', being factual, humorous and also uplifting.

Therefore, on the back of many requests, I found myself sat at my kitchen worktop, coffee to hand, candles on and laptop ready.

I have been asked what my aim was when taking on this gargantuan project, as when I first started to form in my head some kind of order of events and put pen to paper so to speak, the task ahead seemed unreachable. The answer in short was, I didn't really know. Having given it some thought since, I would say it was to offload the things running through my mind and to hopefully help anyone else who finds himself or herself in the same situation, whilst giving some factual references too.

I hope you enjoy reading Mrs H's 'Storm in a D Cup' and in the words of some famous comedian whose name evades me, 'If you like it tell your friends, and if you don't, keep your mouth shut'.

Happy Reading

Mrs H xx

CHAPTER 1
JANUARY 2021

Well, my friends, as that is how I will now think of you, as you will be going on this 'journey' with me. Yikes, I have said it! The journey word that we hear so often on many a reality TV show, usually with some kind of tear-jerking story with sweeping emotional music that pulls at the audience's heart strings. I am only on Chapter 1, paragraph 1 and I've said it already, and I am not even on the X Factor, Britain's Got Talent, or Strictly. Ohh, but everyone loves a journey.

I want to make this more of an adventure, and hopefully, as well as giving you some facts, add some of my humour and personality to lighten the situation. You may be reading this as one of my family, friends or colleagues, or, you may not know me from Adam (whoever Adam is!) but as I keep telling Mr H, I am the funny one in our relationship☺

I have never written a book before. Why would I have? It's not something that I ever planned or thought I would ever do. I love reading, but never ever contemplated putting pen to paper or saw

MRS H'S STORM IN A D CUP

myself as the next Lynda La Plante or JK Rowling. I have many different interests, but not anything really of any substance or what I thought others would be interested in.

Tell you what; it's really hard to even get going. How do you start for instance? Is 'Once Upon A Time' too much of a cliché?

On those nights when I could not sleep with either worry or due to the steroids I had to take, I would lie there thinking of what I would say if I indeed got round to writing anything. I had what I thought were some really good, funny things to say and meant to write things down so I wouldn't forget. Did I do that? No, I didn't! So now I have to rely on the power of recall which when you still have some 'chemo brain' to deal with, and yes, apparently, it is a fact, it is taking slightly longer than anticipated. By the way, I think I will play on that chemo brain thing for some time to come ☺

I asked myself some questions, thinking, was I wasting my time, would anyone really be interested?

Q. Is anyone going to be interested in what I have to say?
Q. Can I remember everything that I want to say?
Q. Can I make any sense of the things going round my head?
A. I don't really know the answer to any of these

questions, but if by reading this, it helps just one person, it will have been worthwhile.

Boy, this is much harder than I thought. I mean, I can put a mean letter together to say a Bank Manager (not that there are any real Bank Managers these days, and if there are, they don't look old enough to even know their times tables), or any other business you may need to converse with, but a book. Come on - get real Mrs H. I even struggled back in the day when you used to send everyone a postcard when you were on your holidays.

Do you remember those days? You would get to your destination of choice, settle in, have a wander round and then you had to make sure you got your postcards sent off asap, as if you didn't, you would be home before them. They would read:

"Having a nice time, weather great, hotel lovely, beach nearby and sea like a dazzling millpond. Wish you were here etc, etc"

Going off at a tangent, which I may do many times whilst writing this epistle, I can remember being on holiday and actually copying what my friend had written on her cards and firing them off to my nearest and dearest. Lazy I hear you say!! Correct.

For the record, I did actually work for a Bank for 24 years so, yes, I do remember real life, stiff upper lipped, scary Bank Managers. Those were the days. Not like now – 'Computer says No' and barely a cashier in sight and don't even get me going on the subject of queue busters, tripping up and down with their Madonna like headsets on.

Throughout those 24 years, I moved branches a few times and made some lifelong friends. If you just stop for a moment and think back to your own history, the memories you have are priceless and you must cherish each and every one of them. I would urge you to stop once in a while, sit back and remember the good times, and the good people.

There are many stories I could tell you about life at NatWest and in particular my time at Oldham, 10 Yorkshire Street Branch. Oh, the Christmas parties we used to have, that usually required some kind of fancy dress attire. One year, one of my besties, Alison and I went as Christmas trees. Her mum, an A Class seamstress, knocked us up these green, A Line tunics with pockets for a battery pack, a hoop at the bottom to give it a tree like effect, baubles sewn all over and full on twinkly lights. I remember having a huge headband with a star on top and green wellies for the trunk. At the end of the night, Alison still looked pristine but I, and I don't know how, looked like the tree surgeon had come along and taken an axe to me.

Like I said, good times.

So where do I start? I suppose I need to introduce myself, so here we go.

My name is Joanne Hinds (formerly Middlehurst and hereon and previous to be known as Mrs H). At the time of writing, I am 58 years old, but by the time I finish, I will be 59 and if I don't get a wiggle on, maybe older. I live in Stalybridge, Cheshire, (ha, a proper Cheshire Housewife and no filler or Botox in sight) with my husband Chris (hereon and previous to be known as Mr H) and my 2 Ragdoll cats, Georgie and Serendipity. Yes, imagine visiting the vets with that one and them shouting, Serendipity Hinds! We also have the most beautiful Maine Coon, Mr Bojangles.

Sadly, and that word does not even cover it, I have had to come back to edit this part as we have since February lost our beloved BoBo and my second skin, Georgie, who had been stuck to my side for 13 years. That cat had a second sense and whilst I was ill, I am 100% convinced he knew and would not let me out of his sight, nestled into my chest and at the side of me most nights. He knew that I needed him.

The memories I spoke about earlier include our furry friends and we will miss them forever. We were and still are both heartbroken and have a huge hole in our lives.

This is the boring bit, but hang on in there, as it gets

better. I could definitely tell you some tales about the first two places of employment (that might be my second book). I left school at 16, having gained a place at Tameside College to do a Medical Secretarial Course. I loved my typewriting lessons, in fact, I won the school prize for typewriting and back then, it was on one of the old manual machines and if my memory serves me correctly, we learnt to type to music. We did however, have one electric machine, though compared to what we are used to today, it looked pre-historic and cumbersome. If you were good, you were allowed to use it and I was lucky enough to have this privilege. If I do say so myself, I can still crack a good few words a minute out.

My mum used to go to work on the bus with a woman whose daughter worked for NatWest. Before I knew it, I had an interview, and was tipping up at NatWest 55 King Street Branch in Manchester. I was 16 and not very worldly wise, in fact, I don't think I had ever even been to Manchester on my own, so this was scary but exciting. It was ever so posh. It had a very strange lift called a 'paternoster' (Google it) which was an open lift that went over and under in a loop, and you stepped in and out of it whilst it was still moving. Can you imagine the 'Health and Safety Police' allowing that these days!

24 years later, I was still there. Well not exactly there, I worked in various branches but never actually in the City centre, more on the outskirts of

Manchester, very down to earth communities with real salt of the earth customers. A great grounding for a young girl who knew nothing. I made many friends along the way who are very dear to me and I love very much.

I took a massive step leaving the Bank, a job I thought I would have until I retired. I just got tired of the constant pressures of sales (though Mr H says I could sell chocolate fireguards and sand to the Arabs). Things had changed massively. Not that I am against change, but sometimes it's not for the greater good. Well that was my opinion. I had already secured my new job before leaving the Bank and went on to do a 16 year stint working for Greater Manchester Police, in various roles and departments and most certainly saw the darker side of life. At least I didn't have to sell anything there. I loved working for the Police and much the same as before, made many wonderful, lifelong friends who are stuck with me.

I would still be there if it had not been for the unit I worked in being re-designed – I will call it that, but it was much more destructive in reality. You probably know the scenario, re-inventing the wheel that is not actually broken, working with the new wheel for a while and then realising the original wheel was actually working alright!! Anyway, it meant that I was going to have to move to a different division and when looking at it logistically, I realised I would be spending too much time travelling for no meaningful gain. I was given the option of Voluntary Redundancy – yehh £££ in the bank. It was a no brainer. This would mean that I could start my slide into retirement too. Happy days.

I still wanted to work, as I didn't feel ready to finish completely and I managed to secure a part time job straight away and am now working for Tameside Council in a small team. Need to try and claw back some of that council tax I pay them every month! I am on my way to retirement, the 'slide has started'.

Both Mr H and I are involved with our Local Hospice – Willow Wood. We throw ourselves into fundraising events and lots more.

That's enough about me, though actually that's not quite true as this book is 'all about me'☺ I really am Mrs Average, just getting on with life and enjoying myself.

That brings me to that day in January 21. I was doing my volunteering shift on the reception desk at Willow Wood and realised that I had not made the appointment for my mammogram check. The letter had been in my bag for a week or so. Naughty.

Phone call made, and they asked if the appointment was for a routine check or was it on the back of the Family History Clinic. I really had no idea, so they had a look and confirmed it was indeed a routine check, as I had been discharged from the FHC. For the record, I was under the FHC due to family history, as the name would suggest. On asking why I had been discharged, they replied 'you are not considered to be high risk'. Brilliant. Appointment made for 8 January 2021. I was pleased if not surprised that my appointment was going ahead so soon, being in the Pandemic and all and people saying that medical appointment were like gold dust.

How lucky was I?

8 January 2021

And so it Begins

Mammogram appointment day and would you believe it, we had at least a foot of snow at 'Hindsy Towers'. Just so you know, we live up 'top of t'hill'. We can have snow when nobody else in Stalybridge has. We are in our own little microclimate. A proper little Narnia. I had to scramble around in the garage to find suitable foot attire and snow gear. Suitable garb located, snow shifted and off I tootled.

The mammogram was being done in one of those temporary mobile caravan like vehicles. If you have not been inside one, they are not very big at all, though it is great that they are available without the need to traipse into a hospital. Well I ask you, have you ever tried to get a bulky snow jacket off, one that goes over your head, in the confines of a room that to coin the phrase 'you can barely swing a cat in', not that I would want anyone to swing any such animal. Well I can tell you now. I felt like flippin Harry Houdini trying to get out of that jacket, you know, the illusionist who wriggles out of a straightjacket with chains round it. I had to bang on the door for the technician on the other side to pull it from my body. Not a good start at all.

The Mammogram

Mammograms are rarely at the top of your 'I can't wait to do list'. If you ask anyone who has had one of these, firstly you get the letter inviting you, with the instruction of what is going to happen.

1. Do not wear deodorant or talc. Well if there is ever a day when you might need it, when you might perspire slightly more than usual, then this is it
2. Wear lose clothing – not a problem
3. You will strip from the waist up and be asked to stand in front of the X-Ray Machine – not nice and a bit embarrassing in a self-conscious kind of way
4. You will put your breast between the plastic plates and stand in a very awkward position. You will then wait whilst the technician

squashes your bosom to within an inch of its life (the letter obviously does not say this) but that's what they do

Imagine putting something the size of say an orange to the size of a small melon (depending on the size of your bosom) into a photocopier then squashing it shut and asking said person to stay still and just relax. Barbaric to say the least. You would have thought that by now they would have found an easier, less traumatic way of doing these tests. But alas, not yet, so squishy squashy it was.

Mammogram over, snow gear back on and trudge back home. Hopefully the results will come through quickly and that will be that.

> ***'Hang on in there – sometimes we have to walk***
> ***through a few storms***
> ***Before we see a rainbow'***
> *(Jane Lee Logan)*

14 January 2021

One week post mammogram. It's a Thursday so I am once again sat doing my volunteer work at the Hospice. Nothing to report. A usual day. That is until I get home.

Mr Postie had been that morning and Mr H had intercepted a letter that looked important and addressed to me. We are not one of those couples who bothers about who opens what post. If he wins big on the lottery or 'Ernie' comes a knocking, I want to know.

Mr H opened the letter that in a nutshell said that there was an irregularity in the mammogram result and that I needed to go for a follow up appointment at the Nightingale Centre in Wythenshawe. The standard letter they send to everyone I imagine. Quite normal to be called back. Not to worry. Happens to X% of patients etc, etc.

Not to worry, that is until you get one of these letters and then you have to be superhuman not to worry.

The appointment was for the following week, but Mr H wasn't having that. Oh no. He didn't want me to have to wait or to have to go through a weekend when I would worry myself sick. He phoned them and by chance, or whatever you want to call it, they had an available appointment the next day.

How lucky was I?

I got home from my shift on that normal day. Mr H sat me down and told me about the letter and his phone call. He knew I would be upset, anxious and whatever other words you want to put to it. He wasn't wrong.

15 January 2021

Appointment No 1: at the Nightingale Centre in Wythenshawe

Ultrasound/Biopsy

Bit of history: Each year approximately 50,000 patients are screened from the Greater Manchester area and 13,000 appointments are made at The Nightingale Centre. A team of dedicated breast care nurses are based at the centre, offering advice and support to patients diagnosed with breast cancer.

The Nightingale Centre offers state-of-the-art diagnostic and treatment services to women and men with breast cancer. Opened in July 2007, the building is located on the University Hospital of South Manchester complex in Wythenshawe.

The Nightingale Centre co-ordinates the NHS Breast-Screening Programme for the Greater Manchester area and provides a base for one of the most ambitious breast cancer research programmes in Europe.

The centre has specially designed consultation, examination, counselling, mammography, radiology, and ultrasound rooms. There are also rooms dedicated to pathology, prosthesis, lymphedema and bone densitometry.

As well as this, The Nightingale Centre is the home to many of the Prevent Breast Cancer researchers and provides training facilities aimed at addressing the shortage of breast cancer specialists.

Basically, I was in safe hands and was going to one of the best places in the country.

We were up early doors as neither of us had a good sleep. Remember though, the letter said that that this was routine and that most patients go forward to have completely normal results.

It had been snowing again up in Narnia, typical, but not too bad, so we were able to slide off the estate without too much trouble. Not much chit chat on the way there, which is not like us at all. Both encased in our own thoughts.

The Nightingale is located in the grounds of Wythenshawe Hospital, Greater Manchester, but on its own site with its own parking. We parked up and when I got out of the car, ours was the only one with snow on the roof. It hadn't even blown off coming down the motorway and people were staring like we had come from the Arctic.

Don't forget we are in the middle of the blasted Pandemic, so Mr H was not allowed to even come into the building with me. I was fine because remember, most tests results are negative. I had nothing to worry about surely, as there were no lumps or bumps or changes in my breasts.

Mr H has a customer that way on so was going to go there and wait for me. We said goodbye. 'Try not to worry' he said. Everyone says that. It's just what people say. Easier said than done, but I donned my mask and in I went.

I am not sure if anyone else does this, but for any hospital appointment, I always like to make an effort with what I'm wearing. Bit like trying to get an upgrade into First Class. Just for the record, I have sneaked into First Class on a train many a time, and got away with it!! Well my dad did do 42 years hard labour for British Rail so I feel it is my birthright. So on this cold, snowy, morning, I had a gorgeous new Karen Millen fur coat on, not real obviously. Yikes, I mean it was not real fur, not that it was a snide KM from down Cheetham Hill!! I had a cosy scarf wrapped tightly round me, and my best leather gloves. Bad choice. I boiled alive whilst I was sat there waiting. Hopsitals are always so hot.

Some more background about the Centre. It was designed following consultation with breast cancer patients and staff. The interior is light and airy, offering a peaceful and welcoming atmosphere for patients. It incorporates a glazed atrium entrance and waiting area with beautiful stained glass. There are planted areas of landscaping, two internal courtyards and a tranquillity garden.

It was all of the above but that day it felt strange. Rows of chairs with notes on every other one saying you could not sit on them. Chevrons on the floor –

screens at the reception desk. This is what had become normal to us – wear a mask, sanitise your hands, keep your distance. It was peaceful but not in a comforting way. There was a tension in the air.

Under normal circumstances, myself and most of the other women there would probably have had someone with us for support. A husband, a mum, a sister, a friend. Not possible. Blasted Pandemic.

Hospitals are normally quite noisy places, but on that day, it was eerily quiet as we were all basically sat on our own. Worry showing in the eyes of many of the patients. Mask wearing meant that we no longer saw faces, just those eyes, staring with worry and concern. It was quiet, no chatter, only thoughts to keep us company.

This theme actually followed most of the appointments I had to attend over the ensuing months. I really wanted Mr H with me. The calm in my storm. My Mr H. I was not naive enough however to think that I should be treated any differently to anyone else. They hadn't picked on me to be on my own, it was the same for everyone. I just had to get on with it.

I sat there waiting. Waiting for that shout of your name is torture. Tick Tock, Tick Tock. A nurse comes out, 'is it me, is it my turn?'. No, not yet. Tick Tock. I need the loo. No. I can't go. What if I miss my turn! I can hold on. I hope they call my name soon. I can't stand all this waiting.

Here she is again. We all look up, listening with anticipation. Mrs Hinds. Yikes, it's me.

Up I get and can you believe it, it was the same technician who had performed the original mammogram in the caravan in Ashton. Remember, the jacket over the head scenario. She remembered me. A familiar face. I was ok. I'd done this before. Off we set to the examination room. She explained that it was almost the same machine as before, but with a little bit more technology so they could look more closely.

It was the right booby that needed to be re-looked at. You know the script. Squishy squashy. In it went. Imagine a stranger, handling your bits. This way, that way. You try not to make eye contact. Up a bit, down a bit, fire. It's like the 'Golden Shot' – you have to be of a certain age to understand that. If you don't know, Google it.

Apparently, I am a perfect patient and do exactly what I am told to do. First part done. She tells me to wait in a different waiting room for the next part of the procedure. An ultrasound and possible biopsy. See that wasn't too bad.

I sit and wait. Same as before. It's so quiet. Tick tock.

Mrs Hinds. Yikes, it's me again. This time I am taken into a relatively small room with an examination bed and another space like machine. The lights are dimmed. Strip to the waist and pop on the bed.

MRS H'S STORM IN A D CUP

There is a nurse and a radiologist. Ultrasound first. These are often done to find out if a problem found by a mammogram is a cyst filled with fluid or a solid tumour. They are not painful or uncomfortable.

She fiddled around with the equipment, backwards and forwards studying the screen and then said she needed to pop out to speak to a colleague. OMG Red Flag. Said colleague came back with her to introduce herself as a Senior Consultant Radiographer. Larger Red Flag.

I now start to panic. On another note, it had been a long time since I had been in such a confined space with three other people and in some way was quite nice, though it would have been better under different circumstances. It felt quite claustrophobic. I was getting hot and clammy.

The Senior then proceeded to perform the ultrasound again. Studying the machine intently. The nurse had hold of my hand. I start to cry. I can't help it. I am scared now.

The Senior asked why I was crying. I know it is something they do day in day out but really. This was not part of my daily routine. Did she really need to ask that question! Could she not see I was scared?

For those of you who do not know me, I had thyroid cancer 15 years ago. I am fine with that, I go for regular check-ups. I have a history of breast cancer in my family and deep down I always thought that it would get me, that I was a ticking time bomb. Don't get me wrong. It wasn't something that was constantly on my mind but every now and then, the Devil on my shoulder would rear its ugly head. I try not to think about the 'what ifs'. It is really hard – you can't help it.

The feeling never really goes away, it's there in the back of your mind but it can appear at any time and mess with your head and your emotions. I try to keep it locked in a box deep in the depths of my mind. Sometimes it's just not deep enough. The physical scars may heal but the emotional ones stay with you. There is no magic wand to get rid of them. The 'what ifs' are always there.

Her response when I told her about my previous history and my fears was, 'Don't worry we can cure you'.

Hang on a minute. I hadn't even had a biopsy or anything yet. What was she saying? Like I said though, this is their bread and butter. They perform these tests every day and looking at that screen, she could obviously tell. Oh no. My heart is racing and my eyes are tearing up.

I will just skim over the next bit. The biopsy. This is a procedure to remove a sample of breast tissue for testing. The sample is sent off to a lab where it is examined to provide a diagnosis. To simplify, they numb the area, stick a probe in to pull out some tissue and that's that. Plaster on, Bob's your Uncle, off you pop.

I was still upset. The nurse was lovely, telling me to try and not worry. It would be ok whatever the outcome. An appointment was duly made for the following week.

I rang Mr H to come and collect me. I got in the car, looked at him and my face said it all. I didn't need to wait for the biopsy result. That Senior had said she could cure me. Why would she say that if it wasn't cancer? Don't get me wrong, I wanted more than anything for it not to be but my gut was telling me otherwise.

I told Mr H everything that had happened. He was obviously upset but always looks at the positives in everything. He says you shouldn't worry until you know you have something to worry about.

That's easy enough surely. That is what I will do!!

Those 7 days were the longest ever. We did not tell anyone, as at that stage there wasn't anything concrete to say. Why worry people unnecessarily. We tried to carry on as normal. At least being in lockdown meant we didn't have to go out and socialise. I've got a bit of a blank for that week. Can't really remember what we did. We obviously were worried but I just kept thinking what that Senior had said. 'We can cure you'. She must know.

The waiting is the worst thing. The examination, the procedures, the scans, the biopsy. The unknown. It is truly terrifying not knowing what you are dealing with.

22 January 2021

Appointment No 2: at the Nightingale Centre in Wythenshawe
Results Day

This was the only appointment that they allowed Mr H to come to. Back down that motorway again. This is getting to be a regular thing. I am safe, Mr H is with me.

Same procedure once we were in the building. Damn COVID. We sit, we wait. Tick tock, tick tock. At least I am not on my own this time.

The nurse appears. Mrs Hinds she shouts. It's our turn.

This time we are actually seeing the Consultant. The main man, a Mr Dimopolous. Into the 'Lion's Den' we go. He is not on his own – there is a nurse with him. Me thinks, not a good sign.

He starts to talk. I hang onto his every word trying to understand what he is saying. He gets straight to the point. I like that. No beating around the bush, straight to the point. My worst thoughts confirmed. It is a cancerous lump.

Oh Shit. Sorry, no bad language alert. Too traumatised. When you hear those words, your world stops for what seems like an age as you try to make sense of what you are being told. I tried to hold back the tears and stared intently at the Consultant. I am clutching Mr H's hand as if my life depends on it. What this man is telling me is actually that. What he is telling me is what I need to make me well and for my life to carry on. Carry on it must. I have too much to live for and so much to do. I am going nowhere.

I try hard to concentrate on what he is telling me. I do not talk. I do not cry. I need to listen. I knew what he was going to say. It is surreal. I try to take note of the details. I must pay attention.

He must think I am a right hard bitch. I have no emotion. I am trying to make sense of what he is saying. I do not speak.

Mr H still has tight hold of my hand and me his. I hear his words but they are just jumbling round my head. I think he is saying that it is a very small lump. I hold on to that. There will be surgery. Good, get it out of me. Radiotherapy to follow. Again, good as I want to make sure everything is gone. He says there is no indication that I will have to have to have chemo. Good. He draws diagrams to explain what will happen.

They were going to take the lump and a margin of tissue around. They would also take some lymph nodes to check that they were clear. Good. Get it out of me. If it is not supposed to be there, be gone. All sounds very simple. I think he was a nice man, though I could only see his eyes. They looked kind. I have to trust him.

He says that he will book me in for the surgery and be in touch. Please let the wait not be too long. We say thank you.

We then move into the next room with the nurse. She introduces herself. She is a Macmillan Nurse.

If there are any words that you do not want to hear, they are:

Cancer – Chemo – Macmillan

Just the word Macmillan fills me with dread. You only have one of these if you are dying.

Let me put that one to bed straight away. This is not the case. I Googled to find out. It says:

Q. Are Macmillan nurses only for terminal cancer patients?
*A. Don't worry too much as **Macmillan may come in at any stage they are needed**. Their role can range from advice and support to newly diagnosed patients through to end of life care.*

Q. What is a Macmillan nurse?

*A. Macmillan nurses are **specialist cancer nurses with experience and qualifications in cancer care**. They can help you to understand your cancer diagnosis and treatment options and support you through your cancer experience.*

There – not too bad then. She is a specialist nurse who will be able to help me understand what is happening. Good.

We sit with her as she starts to go through what the Consultant had just told us. They know from experience that you do not take things in. That your brain goes into a fog situation.

I had been going through the motions and trying to be positive. I can't hold them in any longer. The tears start to flow. I can't breathe. The damn mask does not help. She lets me take it off.

Mr H is upset too. He tries to comfort me. He tries to keep strong but it is hard. I am his wife. His Jo Jo. How can this be happening again?

Language alert!!! Cancer is shit. Watching your loved ones trying to make some sense out of it. Trying to be brave. It is the worst thing ever.

It's not fair – why me again? Mr- H said 'why not you?' which sounds really hard but then he said that it doesn't know it's me, as in his JoJo – because if it did, if it knew who I was and what I am, it would never, ever come near me.

Brave is a word you hear a lot where cancer patients are concerned. It's a strange one. You try and put on a brave face for sure even if it is really some kind of mask, but why would people call you this. It's not like you have a choice. Fire Fighters are brave. The Police are brave. I am not a hero. I am in this position not because I want to be but because I have no choice.

"Life isn't about waiting for the storm to pass... It's about learning to dance in the rain."

(Vivian Greene)

I eventually stop blubbering. We listen carefully to what she has to say. It is easier now, as the initial shock has eased slightly.

Eyes are wiped and noses blown. This is a question for another time maybe, but where does snot come from? I know, gross☺

We are provided with lots of information leaflets, and we now need to go home and process things.

We head home. We are silent. We have a mountain to climb.

The Mountain

If the mountain seems to big today, then climb a hill instead

If the morning brings you sadness, it's ok to stay in bed

If the day ahead weighs heavy

And your plans feel like a curse

There no shame in re-arranging

Don't make yourself feel worse

If a shower stings like needles, And a bath feels like you'll drown

If you haven't washed your hair in days

Don't throw away your crown

A day is not a lifetime

Don't think of it as failure, just a quiet, kind retreat

It's ok to take a moment

From an anxious, fractured mind

The world will not stop turning

While you get re-aligned

The mountain will still be there

When you want to try again

You can climb it in your own time

Just love yourself till then

(Poem by: Laura-Ding Edwards)

We get home. We have people to tell. Oh no. I can't do it. However, they need to know. We are still in a daze. Mr H takes control. He will make the calls. He will know what to say.

The call I dread the most is the one telling my Aunty. She herself had breast cancer a few years ago. She knows the script. She has walked in the same shoes. She is fine. She is a warrior. She only has me. I know how upset she will be.

She answers the phone. Usual telephone chitchat. 'We have something to tell you'. Silence. Mr H relays the situation to her. Don't forget. It is small. They can cure me. We must be positive.

I am sure she is in shock, but tries not to show it. Oh how I wish this was not happening, that I was not having to burden her.

We have the same conversation with Mrs H Snr and my closest friends. It is the same reaction from them all. Shock. They don't really know what to say. What is the right thing to say? We try to re-assure them with the information that we had been given. I can now say that they were all positive and supportive.

I was lucky. This blighter had been picked up early. It was very small and with the treatment plan they had in place for me, everything was going to be ok. It was a waiting game now

Telling my Wider Group of Friends

I decided to bare my soul. Not my breast you will be glad to hear, on my army of friends, family and anyone else who wanted to listen. Baring my breast was something that I would have to do on far too many occasions for my liking.

Of course, it is 2021, so where else can you reach most people but by the great platform we know as 'Social Media'. I sat down and set about how and what I was going to say. I can't lie, it was hard to see the screen as tears blurred my eyes. It was a scary place that I was in, but I wanted to make sure that I pitched my post in just the right way.

During this read, I will quote directly from my Facebook page, so if you have already read it, tuff, read it again☺

From my Facebook page -23 January 2021

I never imagined I would have to write this post, but such is life, and things are sent to try us.

I am not posting this for sympathy or anything like that, but just to let you know that yesterday, I was diagnosed with a small, unwanted lump in my breast, picked up at my routine mammogram, so no actual lump to feel. Thought I was dealing with a 'Storm in a D Cup' but alas this was more like a giant mug.
We have a plan in place to get the blighter out and that cannot come soon enough.

The purpose of this post is to ask you all to pass the message on to your friends and loved ones. If you get that letter to attend for a mammogram or any other test for that matter – DO NOT PUT IT IN THE CAN'T BE BOTHERED DRAWER. You make that appointment and always remember 'If in doubt, check it out'.

I have been lucky in that having no lump to feel,

mine was detected at such an early stage. This is why we have these tests. A bit of discomfort and possibly embarrassment is nothing.

Love to my rock, Chris Hinds, my Mr H, who is always there for me – I now have a list of jobs on the go as I might as well milk the situation.
Early detection saves lives.

Much love
Mrs H xx

> ***'I must have hope – remember, some of the most beautiful things***
> ***Have to move through darkness before they blossom'***

Bearing in mind the situation we were all still in with the Pandemic still prevalent, media reports were flying around saying that hospital appointments, in particular cancer related ones, were being cancelled/postponed.

I am forever grateful that this was not the case for me. I literally had an appointment every week for one thing or another. I was on a rollercoaster, that was for sure.

CHAPTER 2
'MAGSEED'

A week after the diagnosis, I had to go to the Nightingale again to have what they call a 'Magseed' put inside me. Think I forgot to tell you that.

Q. What is a Magseed?
A. A Magseed is inserted into a person with a needle, under local anaesthetic and ultrasound or stereotactic X-ray guidance. It is to help guide surgeons during a breast lumpectomy for impalpable breast cancer. At the time of surgery, Magseed's location is detected with the Sentimag probe (a magnetic sensing system).

My understanding of this was that they would stick this thing inside me so that when the surgeon did his bit, he would have some kind of magnet on the outside to find the exact location. Apparently, the Magseed it is about the size of a piece of rice.

I am back in the waiting room. I am becoming a frequent flyer here. Pity they don't do some kind of reward points! I am sure I would be up for a set of pans by now.

Same old. Sit and wait. Tick Tock.

For some reason, this time, I do not feel quite as anxious. This procedure means that I am one-step nearer to the blighter being removed. Bring it on.

Back into the Ultrasound room. Familiarity. It's not too bad.

You would think you would get used to stripping off in front of strangers. This did not get any easier for me. I hated it. Contrary to what people may think, I am a very private person. Can't stand communal changing rooms or sharing rooms with anyone other than Mr H. Maybe it's something to do with being an only child. Whatever it is. I do not like it.

Tuff. It is what it is as they say. Therefore, it's boob out again. Lie back and relax. What a stupid thing to say. They try to cover you up and give you some kind of modesty but when it comes to it, booby is out for all and sundry to look at, poke and press. I do not like it.

Enter Radiographer stage left. The show is about to start. They try to make small talk with you. Idle chitchat. You try to respond, but when they are coming at you with an implement as big as a knitting needle, it is hard to think of what to say. Only kidding about the knitting needle, that was for dramatic effect only. It's more like a crochet hook!!

Anyway, they fiddle and faff about under ultrasound procedure to try and get this little magnet in. Back and forth. Constantly checking the machine. Let's try again. Flippin eck, they can't find where they are going. More prodding and poking.

Sorry Mrs H, we can't seem to find the right spot as it is so small. Hey, that's good isn't it? We are going to have to try and get it in using the mammogram machine. So back to the waiting room for me again. Tick Tock.

Not too long to wait and they are shouting my name again. It's the same mammogram room I was in a couple of weeks ago. Familiarity. There are two young radiographers. They explain what they are going to do. Basically, they were going to have to clamp me into the machine. Nice. Retreat behind their screened off computer so they could see the X-ray and hopefully insert the seed that way.

Q. Is Magseed insertion painful?
A. The injection may sting for about 15 to 30 seconds. The radiologist then uses a thin, hollow needle to insert a Magseed into the suspicious tissue, guided by additional images. The insertion site is covered with an adhesive bandage. Most women feel pressure or pulling but not pain.

So imagine the scene. Booby needs clamping down in between two plastic plates. Squishy squashy. Looks like a donut having the air sucked out of it. I swear if they had gone any tighter, I would have popped.

I need to breathe, as I know I am holding my breath. If they do not hurry up, they will be dealing with something different altogether. They don't actually know this, but holding my breath is something of a regular occurrence with me. I hold it when I am concentrating hard or say painting my nails. In fact, whilst I am writing this Mr H has just shouted from the next room for me to take a breath. I must really be working hard.

I can honestly say however, that this procedure was not painful at all. Uncomfortable, yes. It took quite a long time, but they needed to be exact with their insertion. They were dealing with minute measurements. Good job I have plenty of patience and am a good patient.

Yehh. It's in. Plaster on. Bob's still your Uncle and ready to go.

There was a bit of bruising over the next few days but nothing really to cause any concern. If you want to know about bruising, that will come later. A proper Crocodile Dundee moment.

What's next? Yikes, surgery. I get my letter. Again, no wait, but what's this? They are sending me to The Spire. The posh Private Hospital. Very nice. I will fit in very nicely there (delusions of grandeur). In reality, it does not really matter where you are as long as the man/woman with the knife knows what they are doing.

'Don't'confuse a difficult chapter with your whole life's story
It might be just that it is time to turn the page to see better things'
(Jane Lee Logan)

From my Facebook page – 6 February 2021

Magseed and Surgery Prep

It has been a while since I updated you on what is going on at Hindsy Towers. The support and love, advice and shared experiences have been phenomenal and I thank you all so much for taking the time to think about me.

I have had beautiful flowers, gifts and cards and I appreciate all the phone calls. They are very much appreciated as it is hard not being able to see people in the flesh for a natter and a brew.

Last week, I was back at the Nightingale Centre, and can truly say that the staff there are all amazing. I had what is called a 'Magseed' implanted into my breast. This is basically a tiny magnet so when they do the surgery, then can find the exact spot. I did not feel a thing but this is possibly because Mr H says that I have skin like a rhino and I am not wired right. He loves me really.

I have had to be careful going past any fridge magnets though or I could find myself stuck to the side of one of Hotpoint's best (other makes are available) – things could get tricky. I have not as far as I know set any alarms off coming out of M&S!

Apparently, this little magnet seed is as effective on day 1000 as it is on the day it is inserted. I am not sure if it is removed during surgery but if not, the next visit through airport security will be interesting. Under normal circumstances, I am usually the one in a group that gets stopped. I'd like to see them try and frisk me!!

We have the date for surgery. Aghh

CHAPTER 3
THE OBLIGATORY COVID TEST

We are going on a 44 mile round trip tomorrow to Trafford General Hospital for a COVID test. Yikes, that's local isn't it! Well, it's a trip out I suppose. Then it is straight into isolation for Mr H and me, ready for surgery day which is next week.

Our World War 3 Bunker, AKA our garage and freezers are suitably stocked with enough food to hopefully see us through the whole week, but we could end up playing freezer roulette so that will be interesting. Ohh choc ice and chips.

Fast forward to Wednesday. I have to be at the Spire Hospital at 0730 hrs – yikes. Anyone who knows me well knows that this is a tall order for sure. I am usually still looking at the back of my eyelids at this time of the day.

Pack an overnight bag with essentials they said, just in case. There are some of you who will be reading this, who can confirm most categorically, that I do not pack lightly. In fact, I find it impossible. In fact, if I do not get a 'Heavy' sticker on at least one of my cases, I feel that I have done myself an injustice. The LV (Louis Vuitton) on wheels will be making an appearance with new PJs and slippers. I might just draw the line at taking my extension reel with me. I can confirm that this is an absolute essential whenever I go anywhere and is almost always, needed. I think most hotel rooms must be designed by men☺

I have decided that when they ask if I have any dietary requirements, I am going to say I always have fillet steak on a Wednesday or failing that cheese and onion pie, my all time favourite. Can't knock a girl for trying!

Fingers crossed, by the end of Wednesday the 'Storm in a D Cup' will be out. That's not good – it's great. A few weeks to recover then wait for the call for the next stage in the 'journey' – oh no, I've said it again.

This will be radiotherapy. Then boosh, gone. I already know of two people who on the back of my last posts have dug their mammogram appointment letters out and had their tests. That is brilliant news, and just what I wanted to highlight. Don't forget the ultimate message 'Early Detection Saves Lives'.

Much love
Mrs H xx

CHAPTER 4
FEELING DISAPPOINTED

From my Facebook page – 9 February 2021 – feeling disappointed

Another little update for you. Slightly fell off the rails. All prepared and mentally ready for the surgery only to get a phone call to tell me it had to be cancelled/postponed due to a broken piece of equipment.

I won't lie, this affected me slightly. I had been building myself up and counting the sleeps. But I am up today, makeup on, hair brushed and hopefully no tears.

New date is set for next Thursday 18th February 2021. Now at Wythenshawe Hospital with a different surgeon. It is now with a Mr Dave (pronounced Dar Vay). We are out of isolation again, not that it makes a difference as not going anywhere, apart from, yes, you have guessed it, another road trip to Trafford General for another COVID test, and possibly another 'big shop'.

I have even taken my nail polish off, so that will be

going straight back on. At least it gives me more time for Mr H to do 'me roots'.

Disappointing to say the least but as I have said before, these things are sent to try us.

I feel like I am doing the tour of Greater Manchester Hospitals: Tameside, Wythenshawe, Trafford and then hopefully Oldham for the radiotherapy. I feel like a mystery shopper. Well I can report they are all amazing and are getting five star ***** reviews.

That's all for now

Much love
Mrs H xx

CHAPTER 5
THE ACTUAL COVID TEST

In the last few years, these tests have become part of our lives. Lateral Flows, PCRs. Yuk. I am sure that you have seen those test sites that say 'Results in 20 Minutes' – well I can tell you it takes me more than 20 minutes to gear myself up to even start doing my own flippin test.

I don't know about you, but for me they have never gotten any easier. My very first ever PCR was horrendous. Firstly, on reflection, I do not think it was wise of me to have a couple of mouthfuls of tuna/mayonnaise & sweetcorn just before I performed said test. Obviously, I did not realise that at the time.

Mr H was doing his in the kitchen and said that I would probably find it easier if I looked in the mirror to do mine. So, that is what I did. Test stick at the ready. Open wide – ahh. I can't do it. I'm going to be sick. It's not even in my mouth yet. Come on Mrs H you can do it. Ten seconds, they are having a laugh surely. In it goes. Jeez, out it comes. Breath. Compose yourself. In it goes, into the black hole of my mouth. I'm doing it. Yehh. Oh no. I'm gagging and it's only been in about 2 seconds. No way on this earth can I do 10 seconds. I try again. It's like the aeroplane heading towards the child's mouth, encouraging them to eat. Yeh right. It's nothing like that. It's a deadly stick that is about to scratch the back of my throat and inflict some kind of pain on me. You are right. I am such a baby.

Right. I pull myself together. This test has to be completed one way or another. I stand open mouthed determined that I am going to be able to get at least 3 seconds, yes, that is what I am aiming for. I will whip it round quickly and that will be that.
Third time lucky. This time. I am feeling confident, well a little bit. I will do it quickly. That will be the best option. Might even do a quick 3 seconds in 2 if that is possible. Right, mouth is open, stick is in, it's touching the back of my throat. Oh no – I am well and truly gagging. I'm going to be sick. I run to the sink and indeed sick is what I was. That's when I realised I definitely should not have had that tuna. It looked like something the cat would eat. Well not my pedigree puddies. They eat something far more appetising.

Well I definitely am not going to put that implement in my mouth again so up the nose it goes. Yuk, tuna is much better when you eat it than when you sniff it.

Well you can guess what the result was when it came

back. Inconclusive. Traces of fish and sweetcorn detected. Only kidding – negative. So in case you have to do one and struggle like I do, just put the stick in a tin of John West (other products are available).

You can imagine therefore how I was feeling when I tipped up at the Hospital for my test. I duly advised the nurse that I did not have good history doing the PCR test. "No problem" she said. When you open your mouth "Sing". She was surely having a laugh. But no. She said that this would work and that it would be easy peasy – well she did not actually say those words but that is what she meant. So I sang. A long high ahhhhh. Stick was in, touched the side and out. All done and no gagging or sick. Piece of cake. In the words of Jim Royle '10 seconds My Arse'.

I have consequently tried this each time I have had to do a PCR and it does actually work. Got some strange looks when having to do a test in one of those tent things. But hey, I am sure it was better than me throwing up all over the shop.

So If you ever have to do one, think of me trilling at the top of my voice and give it a go.

COVID test is clear. Full steam ahead. Surgery day looms nearer and I pack my back again. It is worse this time. I have to be there by 0700 hrs.

CHAPTER 6
SURGERY DAY & BRA BUYING

SURGERY DAY – 18 February 2021

From diagnosis to surgery was exactly 34 days. How fantastic was that. I could not complain at all about the speed in which I was being projected through the various department and hospital systems. God bless the NHS.

I asked Mr H what were his feelings on that cold February morning:

His reply was simple - helpless. He could not do anything but drive me to appointments and be there for me in whatever way he could.

For the record, he would drive me to the ends of the earth but this is one place that he wished he didn't have to take me.

We were up early. Yes, me, up early, again. I could not sleep anyway. I just wanted to get there and get it over.

The motorway was empty and in darkness. We drove in silence just listening to the early morning radio. The odd word here and there.

I was not scared of surgery. I have had quite a few over the years. There is always that doubt in the back of your mind though that something will happen whilst you are 'under'. 'What if I don't wake up?' 'What if this is the last time that we see each other!' We don't speak of such things.

Wythenshawe Hospital is massive. It is not somewhere that I am familiar with, so that was about to be my first hurdle. We pulled up at the door and Mr H gets the LV out of the boot. We go to the front door but that is as far as he can go. There is a security guard on the door. Jeez, what's that all about?

We say our goodbyes. I am trying to be brave and not cry. The tears trickle down my face and I try to brush them away. I don't want Mr H to worry, even though he will.

'Don't worry Mr H – A few Tears in my Tutu will not stop me dancing'

I am in possession of my 'Pre-Operative Information Leaflet' – it tells you to think about the clothing you will wear to go home in! They don't realise that I think about what clothes I wear to empty the bins (that is a slight exaggeration as I don't actually do the bins!) I had a near miss with one once, when the weight in it nearly transported me down into the garden next door. Very dangerous activity. That is why I let Mr H do them.

Loose fitting clothes with a front fastening is what they recommended. A well supporting, non-wired bra – well I would need to go and buy a few of these. I will come to what happened when I did so, in a little while.

Discomfort and Pain – to be honest, I think this was a given. Found it quite bizarre that the recommendation was to take your own pain relief with you! Must be the sign of the times.

You must not drive yourself home. Would anyone actually even contemplate this? Possibly but what do I know, but I feel sorry for anyone who finds themselves in that position.

Bra Buying

I will tell you now about the bra buying saga. I won't say the name of the store (I think it used to be sponsored by a Saint ☺), but I am sure many of you have purchased from them and had your bazookas measured there. Damn COVID meant that I could not even try anything on or have one of their fitters do my measurements and give advice. I think I must have been back and forwards half a dozen times with badly fitting items.

I went up and down the aisles looking at all the pretty things hanging up. Not for me today. I needed something less attractive, something that would be functional and supportive. I have never actually noticed before, but there was a section for 'post-surgery'. Just standing there in front of these items brought a huge lump to my throat. That sign, for all to see - 'post-surgery'. I still cannot believe that this is happening and that I am in this position. But I will not cry. Not for sure in the middle of a store. Someone might see me.

In fairness to them, the selection they had to offer, whilst not massive was quite acceptable. I made my selection and joined the queue to pay. This is where I feel they let me down. Not on purpose, but none the less, a lesser more fragile person could have crumbled at that pay desk.

In front of the rest of the queue and rather loudly, the cashier asked me if I realised I had picked up a **'post-surgery' bra**? It may have been my state of mind at that particular time, but I thought that this was a rather insensitive thing to say. I did not want to make a fuss so just answered that yes, I knew. I was really quite angry. This was my surgery. This was private to me. I did not want it to be brandished to all and sundry. I know that it was nothing to be ashamed of but it would become public knowledge in my time, when I decided.

I went home and when mulling over what had happened, I decided that the next time I visited said shop I would have a word with someone. Not to get anyone into any kind of trouble, but to just to say that maybe they needed to re-address what they say to customers in similar positions. That maybe they needed to add something into their training. I even had some dialogue ready to share with them, things that I thought would be much softer and caring.

For example:

- *How pretty is this bra, I would imagine it would be really comfortable after surgery!*

- *Not sure if you know, but you don't pay VAT on post-surgery bras, so I will put that reduction through the till for you now.*

The surgery word is still being used, but in a lesser invasive way, letting you know that if by chance you had picked the wrong thing up, great, you would be alerted. Plus, I had no idea until doing some research that you got discount on post-surgery items. Everyone loves a bargain.

The supervisor fully agreed with what I had to say, apologised and said that she would definitely be addressing matters with her staff and any future training.

That's all I wanted, so in the future, nobody is made to feel worse than they already do.

Off on a Tangent about Bras Now

Now, women of a certain size in the bazooka department will know that getting a lovely, pretty, sexy bra to fit is almost impossible. You usually end up with something quite plain (though things are improving). Probably designed back in the day by Isinbard Kingdom Brunel (in case you don't know, he designed suspension bridges)☺

Ha, I am now going to add a tangent within a tangent. On holiday in Turkey one year, one of my besties who is also blessed in the chest department, had one of her bras taken out of her room. Not good, but we always have to find humour in every situation. Firstly, we were on the lookout for anyone with similar sized mammary glands, for surely that would be the culprit. Secondly anyone needing to carry a large amount of, well anything. But the laugh came whilst we were all lying on our sunbeds and above, like a phoenix in the sky, a lonesome parasailer came into our vision. Mystery solved. They obviously needed a new parachute or whatever they use for this particular watersport, and the missing bra was obviously just the ticket☺ We had a good laugh at that.

Again, larger chested ladies will also recognise these traits. Well I hope so, as I cannot believe it's only me who does this kind of thing. I use my bra for lots of things, and yes, when it is being worn:-

- It looks after my credit card if I am in a rush and don't want to take a bag out with me – bit awkward sometimes when you have to go fishing down your top for said card in the middle of Tesco
- I nearly always have a paper hanky stuffed down the middle of my chest – with my history of sneezing I have to be ready at all times
- It is a safe hidey hole for money too – safest place as nobody will find it there
- Pen holder, though you have to be careful with this one
- And I cannot take the credit for this one, but back in my NatWest days, a colleague who had a gargantuan chest, actually put the safe keys down there ☺
- Phone carrier - there is actually no evidence to suggest that carrying your mobile phone down your bra will do you any harm. I personally am not prepared to take the

- chance though.
- To conclude, if I ever get a bit peckish, I can usually find some kind of food item hanging around – I know, gross.

Funnily enough, I was out at weekend in Costa, enjoying my 'frothy, grande, thick and creamy chocolatey, sweet and buttery, smooth cappuccino coffee' – not really, it was a flat white but it sounds good, when I felt a hard pea like lump in my breast. Not that I was feeling myself up in public, merely leaning on the table. Panic. I did nothing more than start delving around and to my relief, said lump moved when I pushed it. Nothing to worry about, I would deal with it later. Said lump turned out to be a peanut that must have fallen out of my mouth and into the abyss of my chest. Did I eat it? What do you think? ☺

'Remember it is ok to take sugar, but keep the lumps out of your cups'

The Males of the Species

Whilst we are on the subject of bras, I thought it would be rude not to take a look into how the male of the species approach purchasing said items. If then by any chance there are any guys reading this book, firstly, I thank you and secondly, take note.

If you have not have had the pleasure of purchasing the obligatory, though usually tacky valentine/Christmas/birthday lingerie, you would not be prepared for the grilling you are given whereby the assistant needs to know the sizing of said garment you wish to purchase.

The perfect bra has to have it all - the shape, the size, the beauty and the comfort. It's such a shame therefore, that perfection is so rare to come by. We absolutely understand that for somebody purchasing said garments on our behalf, this can be a tall order. Leeway is given.

Ladies will probably have witnessed such an event, watching some geezer nervously twitching and checking to see if anyone is watching. God forbid if whilst lurking round the ladies underwear department they should see anybody who knows them. What will they think? The assistant asks what size is required and in response, you they will most probably hold their hands up to demonstrate, looking like they are testing oranges or larger in some cases. She will ask about the cup size, explaining that this is the description for the size of the 'bosom holders'. She will tell them about the cup, the sizes available in the range they are looking at and in a panic, a random letter is most probably just picked out of the air, any letter, the first letter that pops into their head. 'D' Yes that sounds like a good letter. That's what will be chosen, what they will go for. Selection duly made, a swift exit and the said item will be gifted on the relevant day and if you are lucky, it will not still be in the bag it was purchased in but tastefully wrapped and presented.

We can however tell you now. Most of them do not fit. We try them on and wiggle and squeeze into them the best we can so as not to hurt feelings. They are that tight we cannot breath. The overhang looks like something in a butcher's shop window. The wire sticks in threatening to stab us in the heart. We thank you anyway. They will probably come out for an airing once or twice and will then be relegated to the back of the drawer.

Well my friends, I realise we are talking about the 'Storm in a D Cup', but for the record, I was dealing with more of a FF situation!!! 'Flippin Fabulous '.

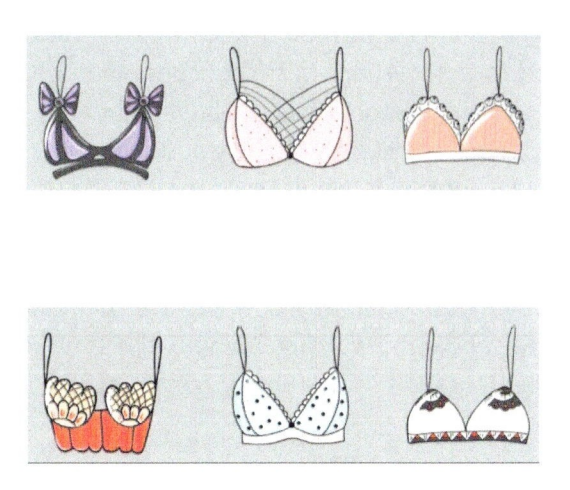

I really did go off piste there, so I apologise and let's get back to the subject in hand.

In case you have forgotten where we were up to, I was just about to enter the hospital. Paperwork in hand and mask on. I entered the building, with the solitary Security Guard on duty, turning to watch Mr H make his way back to the car. Watching him disappearing into the distance is not an image I wish to see again. I was the one having the surgery, but, it was Mr H who looked like he had the weight of the world on his shoulders. I hate to see him upset. His head is down. He is trying to be strong. He is my rock. He needs to be strong. He is my everything. I am his JoJo. I know, slushy, but I don't care.

I am on my own now. I mean I am really on my own. The corridor looms before me, grey and dismal. Unfamiliar. It was surreal. The only time that I had stepped foot anywhere in this hospital was way back in the process, when I had to have a heart scan to make sure my ticker was in good working order. There was not one single solitary soul in sight. I clutched my letter and the instructions telling me where to go. It seemed such a long corridor with no end in sight. I constantly checked the directions on the letter and kept walking. Why is there nobody to ask? The LV rattled along the corridor behind me.

This in itself is strange. Me, carrying my own luggage. I mean, come on. I know some of you think that Mr H carries me and does everything for me. Well not quite everything. He does however move my feet away from the fire if they are burning! Ha ha, got you, we don't have a fire ☺

For many years, we were lucky enough to have BUPA, and the other surgeries I have had have been courtesy of the best private hospitals in the area. You check in and someone takes your luggage to your room. Nice. You trip along to said room and settle in. It's like a hotel room. You turn the TV on. It says hello to you, even knowing your name. What's for tea. That is a very important thing to me as I am always ready for something to eat after having anaesthetic. Well at any time really which is why I am back at Slimming World, again!! Alas though, this is not the case now. Our circumstances have changed, for the better I must add, but to cover me with BUPA is just too expensive. It would be like trying to get insurance on some old, irreplaceable relic. Actually, that is probably a good description of me.

We are not worried though. The NHS gets bad press, sure enough, but they were looking after me like a precious cargo. Wythenshawe Hospital in actual fact has a very good reputation in many areas of medicine and indeed breast surgery I found out was one such area. In fact, my great friends Janet & Neil have a nephew who is a breast surgeon and Wythenshawe is one of the places he would like to work. Ian, in fact was another member of my elite band of trusted advisors. I spoke to him on a number of occasions to ask for his advice and to just check if what I was feeling was normal. I do, however, remember Ian as a wee lad. I am sure he is a wonderful surgeon, but I am glad he was not mine. It would have felt slightly weird having to bear all in front of him.

Back to that corridor. I see someone heading towards me. Fantastic. They might be able to throw some light on where I should actually be heading, as God knows, the directions are not very good. Mind you, I am one of those people who if going by car to a new place, expect the signs to start and the end of my drive and I have no perception of north or south. On that day though, it may be that I was not concentrating as I should have been and can admit now, that I was feeling anxious.

Brilliant, she works at the hospital and knows the lay out like the back of her hand, or so she said. I looked at her hand and there were definitely no corridors or lift signs on them. Still, she points me in the direction I should be heading and off I pop. Where does that saying come from – like the back of your hand? You would get nowhere fast if you looked at mine. Very freckly and increasingly wrinkly. Note to self – I must do something about that.

I am here. I have found the correct Department. It is

dark and very quiet, well it is still so very early. I approach the solitary nurse sat behind the desk, head down, and probably tired, as it will soon be the end of her shift. She smiles. She looks kind. She checks my letter and directs me to a large, airy but empty room. The chairs are located all around the outside of the room. I have the pick of the crop as I am the first there. Who knows how many other women will descend on me.

There is a television in the corner of the room so I pick a seat ensuring that I will have a good vantage point. The sun is coming up. The day is dawning. I settle down and set out my stall. I have my phone, a couple of magazines, a reading book and a puzzle book. I am not allowed anything to eat or drink so no goodies to be seen. Why is it that when you cannot have something, you really, really want it?

I feel quite calm to be honest. Slightly anxious, but now I am here, I just want them to get on with it. I take control of the TV remote. Think I will go for ITV at this stage, but if Holly and Phil get on my nerves, they will be swiftly exterminated.

Two other women join me. They too settle themselves down. We exchange nods and smiles. We are captivated with our own thoughts and worries. We chat a little, exchanging our stories. All three of us have breast cancer, all three stories and procedures were different.

Back to the silence and the hum drum of the TV. Time is ticking but not much is happening. Still not met this Mr Dave character. I need to check him out. Does he have kind eyes? This has become something of a thing with me. As we have all been wearing our masks, the eyes are the only things that we see. They really identify us. Kind eyes to me simply mean that you care. You care about yourself and you care for those you meet.

The first lady is called through and gathers her belongings, trudging off. We wish her luck. It is still only very early. Jeez, I feel like I have been up for hours. I have been up for hours. I am trying to read my book but seem to keep reading the same lines over, and over again.

It is the same waiting game as before. Tick Tock. It is different this time. There is more apprehension, the fear of the unknown. There is more at stake. A nurse pops her head in and shouts for me. Yikes is this it. Is it my turn? In a word, no. We go to a little side room and but her role is merely to go through the admin. Usual, checking of details to make sure you are who you say you are. No, I am someone else, I just thought I would come along for a laugh! Sarcasm at it's best – but did you know that sarcasm is the lowest form of whit but the highest form of intelligence. I am so clever ☺ Obviously, I did not say this outloud, just that devil voice in my head. During the day I am asked this question many times. At least they are making sure and being vigilant.

She explains what is going to happen and then pops the hospital wristband on me. This shit (sorry) is getting real now. The last time I had any kind of band round my wrist, I was in a very exclusive 5* hotel! As long as the service here was 5* I didn't really care.

I am ushered back to the waiting room to await the next stage. It is not too long a wait. I am called back into a different room where there are two Radiographers from I think the Nuclear Science Department – yikes, that sounds a bit, well a lot scary. Now this is where I cannot quite remember the reason why they did what they did. All I know is that yet another needle was stuck into me with something or other in it that I didn't really know the content of. Think it was some kind of dye so the surgeon could find the lymph nodes easily. It didn't hurt. I am all about thing's not hurting.

Ask Mr P, my dentist. I even have to have some kind of stuff rubbed on my gums, probably a light anaesthetic, before I let him perform even a scale and polish. I know. Such a baby.

Going Off on a Tangent

Going off on that 'tangent' again, when I had the

thyroid cancer all those years ago, the treatment I received was 'Radioactive Iodine'. It still bewilders me that what made me better can be so dangerous to others.

I must just mention another dear friend of mine, Helen Evendon (Langford) who I have known since I was a little girl. She also had a similar kind of Thyroid Cancer to me, and I am pleased to say that she is also, many years later, still doing really well.

This is why it is so important for research to continue the way it has done, in order that future generations will be cured.

Back to the treatment I was given. It was all very James Bond. Two chaps from the Nuclear Science Department tipped up, very Blofeld like but minus the cat. I almost quoted the iconic line 'I've been expecting you Mr Bond'!, but I don't suppose M ever greets Bond with her PJs on☺ They had a huge lead briefcase that was padded inside, and the said treatment was literally a single solitary 'Tablet' sat in the middle on it's lonesome. Down the hatch and that was it – I was radioactive – untouchable.

This treatment came well after the surgery and it meant me having a few days at 'The Mother Ship – The Christie'. I was in a room on my own, with an en-suite – very nice. But that was where the nice ended. Not that the treatment was painful, or made me poorly, but I was more or less in total isolation for the whole time. How weird, that in the last few years, millions of people all over the world have experienced feelings of isolation. It wasn't too bad, I had books and a TV, though the nurses only came to see me to deliver my food over the top of a lead screen!!

I was allowed visitors, but they could only be in the room with me for 15 minutes at a time, and they had to sit in the corner behind the lead screen and come nowhere near me. I believe my friends queued up in the corridor waiting their turn. Mr H, rebelled slightly. He came in first then went to the back of the queue for another turn.

When I got home, the isolation continued. We were fortunate enough that we had 2 bathrooms and enough bedrooms for me to have my own. They even said that if we had adjoining rooms, the headboards should not be back to back. Jeez, what was this stuff doing to me? I can tell you what it was doing. It was making sure that any remaining 'C Word' cells, would be obliterated to give me the gift of life.

I had to have my own cutlery, plates, cups etc. Mr H was allowed to cook for me, but not me for him. Yet another benefit I hear you say.

I could not have any visitors in the first week and

then the restrictions reduced each week. No visitors with children. I was literally radioactive. You could have stuck me in the corner like a Christmas tree. I even resorted to talking through the post box to Mr Postie. I literally needed an 'unclean' sticker on the front door!!

Back to the Present Day

Ok, back to the subject in hand, as I am returned once again to the waiting room. It's Holly and Phil time so it must be past 1030 hrs by now. I settle down and make myself comfortable. I've purloined a footstool, so really making myself at home now.

I am just getting settled and they shout me again. A different room. What this time? Well, it is time to meet the other 'Main Man'. Mr Dave. Don't forget how you need to pronounce this, (Dar Vay). In he comes. First impressions – not very tall (possibly a heightist comment but an observation non-the-less), but then again I am sat down. As long as he can reach me on that operating table without the need of an orange box. Nice suit. Very important. In fact, Mr H has one the very same colour. Don't remember him having a tie on, but if he did have, it would have had to be a 'Windsor Knot'. My dad taught Chris very early on in our relationship how to do a 'proper' tie and if I do say so myself, he always looks the dogs doo dah's (notice how I did not use the word that you may think I was going to) when suited and booted. I cannot be doing with sloppily tied ties. Shoes. Now this is also very important. You can definitely tell a lot about a man by looking at his shoes. Very nice. Brown, which is very on trend at the moment, and went with his suit very well.

Going off the subject slightly, when I first met Mr H, his shoes left a lot to be desired, but I gave him the benefit of the doubt. I can confirm that with the benefit of my wisdom he realised the error of his ways and now has a splendid display of extremely nice footwear.

Anyway, getting back to Mr Dave. Introductions made. He was as you will imagine, sporting his hospital mask. Yes, I could see his eyes and they looked ok. Nevertheless, I really wanted to see the face behind the mask. I wanted to see if he looked kind. If he cared. If he smiled.

Can you imagine his surprise when I said 'Right, as you are going to be looking at my boob, it is only fair that I see what you look like. I want to make sure you have a kind face – so drop your mask'. It was a bit like an episode of the Masked Singer – Take it Off, Take it Off. He started to laugh. Bet he hadn't been asked to do that before.

He obliged and the mask was removed - I was happy. He did have a kind face. He could continue.

He went through what was going to happen, though he could not give me a definite timeline, only that out of the three of us, I was to be the last. Flip. Time was ticking on so heavens knows what time I will be done. He ended the conversation with the usual line that you hear on the hospital TV programmes. They always say it 'See you in Theatre'. Don't know why they say this, because by the time the surgeon rocks up the patient is normally well away with the fairies. For all we know, it could be the porter doing the surgery.

I have since learnt that they take the more serious cases into theatre first in case there are any complications. That made me feel better that I was a humdrum, routine lumpectomy patient. Not sure if I have mentioned it yet, that was the procedure that I was going to have, along with some lymph node removal.

I Googled it and it said 'A lumpectomy is a common but major surgery' – In this instance and this instance only, I did not mind being common ☺

Back to the waiting room. It is Loose Women time now, so we are hurtling towards lunch. God, I am hungry. They actually decided that I could have a small amount of water which was nice of them, as my mouth felt like the bottom of a budgie cage. Not that I have tasted the bottom of many budgie cages but you know what I mean.

The second lady had gone when I got back and I am now on my 'Jack Jones' again. It's ok though. Soon be my turn. I have my phone so I am keeping in regular contact with Mr H. It is hard for him too, sat at home not knowing what is going on and where I am up to.

The nurse appears again and this time has the rather fetching hospital gown slung over her arm. It's time to get ready, so let's get this show on the road.

Into the cubicle I go. Well, have you every worn one of those gowns? Bloody awful. The first hurdle is remembering which way round to put them on. Do you have your front bits on show to the world or your backside peeking out? Seem to think it is the latter. I've got me big knickers on though and won't be taking them off for anyone.

They also provide me with some very sexy, bottle green compression socks. There is not a stylish way on this earth that you can wear these I can tell you. They look like they are small enough to fit a child for starters and you then have to fight with them, rolling them up your legs like you are making sausages. They are that tight that I was sure that the skin on my calves would end up on my thighs, and God know there is quite enough there to start with.

I am ready. I sit with my feet up on my stool, fully gowned up with my fluffy slippers on. Come on, I am ready. Nothing. Absolutely nothing happens for what seems like an age. Every time I heard footsteps on the corridor, I thought they were coming to get me. But alas, no.

There is not much to tell you for the next few hours. Yes, flippin hours, as it was just me, myself and I. The only bit of excitement was when a couple of Polish electricians came in to fix a light fitting. Not much interaction there, in fact absolutely none.

It is about 1500 hrs now. I had been sat there, give or take a few trips to different rooms, for what is for most people, the expanse of a working day. I am a patient person but I was starting to get a bit twitchy and worried. Have they forgotten me? What if the surgeon runs out of theatre time? Does that actually happen? Bit like a long distance lorry driver or bus driver!

Eventually the nurse comes in to tell me it is time. I am relieved, as I just want it over now. They took my bag and phone off me, saying that it would be waiting for me on the ward that I would be going to after the operation. I didn't even have time to check in with Mr H to let him know I was on my way. Oh no ☹ What if something happens to me during the operation and I never get to speak to him again. The mind does some terrible things.

It was weird, as I had to walk to the operating

theatre, in my ever so fetching gown, but as the hospital did not seem to be too busy, we did not pass anyone on the way there. Even that seemed surreal. At least nobody would be subject to a view of my rear end.

Once I got there, I was asked all my details to check once again I was who I said I was – well of course I was. Who in the right mind would find themselves stood outside an operating theatre pretending to be someone else!

I am up on the 'table' now. People are buzzing around getting on with their own jobs, their part of the procedure. It all gets a bit heavy then. Pads and stickers attached – oh no I have to take my glasses off. This is when I tell them that I can't see a flippin thing and that my brain does not work without them either. They assure me that they will be very careful with them and they will be at my bedside when I awake. They tape my rings up because there is no way on earth they are coming off – they will have to cut my fingers off to get to them. Which technically, whilst I am 'out for the count' they possibly have the equipment to do such a dastardly task.

The anaesthetist shuffles in. A lovely lady who made me feel at ease, or as at ease as you can be in such a situation. I vaguely remember them putting the blood pressure machine on my arm as it felt really tight and started to hurt, then I can barely remember anything else. Not even the countdown to 'sleepy time'. I am one of those weird people who quite like that feeling you get when being put to sleep. I know, strange.

So that was that for an hour or so. Obviously nothing to report as not aware of anything. Can't even tell you if I had any good dreams.

It's that tangent again ☺ A couple of weeks later I was reading a book and the back cover had the following picture. It really made me belly laugh (I have to admit, at that time I had more belly than I would have liked), and it made me think that I had definitely been in too many hospital scenarios, because I thought the tin cans on the back of the car were heart monitor stickers ☺

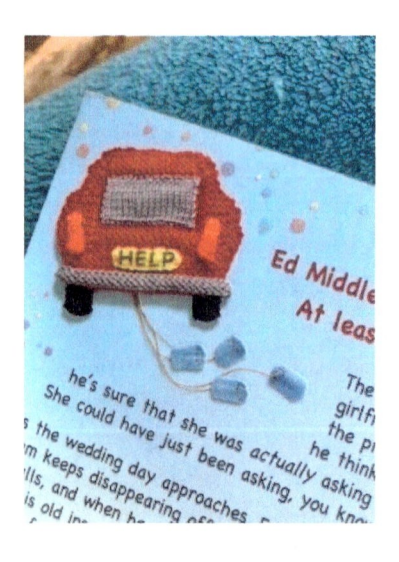

I woke up in the recovery room and felt remarkably fine. A bit woozy and obviously blind (no glasses yet) but apart from that, I don't remember feeling too bad. Oh yes, hungry. That's nothing new. I am not one of those people who cannot eat after a General Anaesthetic, in fact, I can eat almost anything, anytime. That's probably why I am as I have previously said, I am at Slimming World, yet again. I have hit that 'Target' more times than Eric Bristow.

I was wheeled to the ward where I was re-united with the 2 ladies from earlier in the day, my rucksack and my glasses. Yehh, I can see again. There was a lovely male nurse looking after us but for the life if me I cannot remember his name. For the benefit of this read, I will call him Mark! (that's Mr H's middle name). I think I had a bit of a snooze but you can't sleep for long in a hospital and Mark was back and forth doing my observations.

Food, that's what I need now. Mark was duly summoned and I asked could I have something to eat and drink. Oh, if only it had been that BUPA hospital I should have been in, I could have been feasting on fillet steak and chunky chips, displayed in an arty farty jenga type of pattern, but alas no. Off Mark trotted to return with what was actually a veritable feast. I was on fruit juice, a ham sandwich on white bread – yes healthy, hospital, white bread – and quite generously stuffed with ham too. A couple of packets of ginger biscuits a yogurt and a big mug of tea. Heaven.

I think I may have had some kind of a drip attached to me but that was quite quickly removed, allowing me to dispense of the hospital gown that I had become attached to, and I was allowed to put on my own PJs. This was the first time that I had a look at said 'boob'. It actually did not look too bad, just two lots of padding, one where the lump had been and the other where they had taken the lymph nodes. Still looked like it was the same shape as before. I knew I would end up with some scarring but I hoped it would not be too bad. Historically, I have good healing skin so hoped that that this would be the case this time. I have that many scars on my body, it looks a little like a roadmap.

I don't care though. As long as I am ok and they have got everything out.

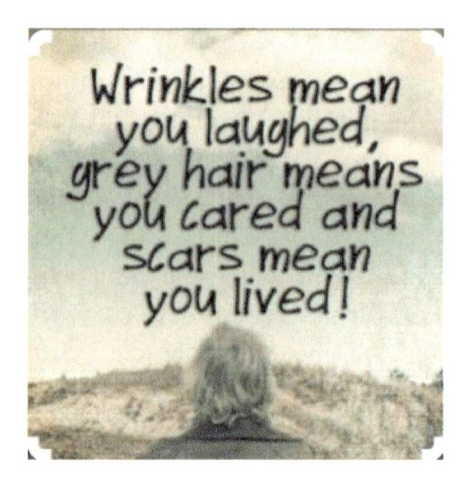

> Wrinkles mean you laughed, grey hair means you cared and scars mean you lived!

One by one the other ladies were allowed home, having stayed for their allotted time after their procedure. That left little old me again on my own. It's a good job I like my own company. By this time it was quite late and I realised I had not phoned Mr H. He would be beside himself with worry.

Indeed he was. He had rung earlier to find out how I was and was put through to the ward, but at that time I was still down in theatre. He then heard nothing for what seemed like hours. By this time, the reception had shut and he could not get through and he did not have the number for the ward. In desperation, he phoned the Nightingale Centre and explained the situation but they did not know the number of the ward either. Panic.

Being the nerd he is, he searched online and found a phone number that was actually the Director's Suite, promptly answered by the HR Director of the Hospital. Yikes. Nothing like going to the top. She was really helpful as one would expect, and said she would find out where I was and more importantly, how I was. She rang back to confirm that I was in recovery and everything was fine. By this time it was almost 1830 hrs. At the same time, Mr H had been fielding calls from everyone asking how I was. Flippin eck, stressful or what whilst I was sat having a picnic.

Meanwhile back at the ward, I asked when I would be going home, as all my observations were fine. But guess what, you can't go home till you've had a wee. Oh no. Anyone who knows me, will tell you that I am like a camel and very fussy about whose toilet I will use. In fact, I very rarely go to the loo when I am out and about, and if I do, it has to be a dire emergency. I can confirm, I have never had a pee in a field or any such place!! However, there are two places, three at a push that if such an emergency occurs, I will go, one being Housing Units, which is a really nice Department kind of store near where we live, and M&S and John Lewis. Funnily enough, all said places usually end up costing us more than the said 'penny' and tend to end up with some kind of food being consumed.

By this time, I have had another mug of tea so my bladder was actually showing signs of bursting. Mark said he would escort me to the loo in case I was a bit wobbly on my feet. He checked would I be ok going into the loo on my own and in horror, I told him that under no circumstances was he coming in with me. I won't even let Mr H look at my wee. It gets worse, as I was then given one of those grey hat like things to perform into. I had no choice. I had to do 'it' or I would have to stay there forever.

Well I can tell you, do it I did. It was like listening to the Co-op horse (you must pronounce it Quorp - I am not quite sure if that is a Northern saying) but you get the gist. I apologised profusely to Mark, though I am sure that he had seen worse.

Mark was due to finish his shift and handed over to the night staff. I must add that all the staff were fabulous and I have nothing negative to say about them or my brief stay at their facility.

Mr H now knew that I was ok and had been told that he could come and collect me. By this time it was gone 2200 hrs. The Hospital was still like a ghost town. That quietness from earlier in the day carried on into the night. They let him come up to the ward to collect me, which was nice, though the nurse insisted on pushing me in the wheelchair. I still had my PJs on but thought, to hell with it, if anyone sees me they would just think I was blending in with the locals (bit controversial but actually again, observational)!

It was so good to see each other. It had only been a day, but seemed like a lifetime. I had been dropped off at 0640 hrs and we did not get home until the next day at 1215am. Now to recover and see what the next step would be.

CHAPTER 7
FEBRUARY 21

From my Facebook page – 21 February 2021

The operation went well and I have two corking bruises to prove it that would put you off your tea for sure.

I was treated to a ham butty courtesy of Wythenshawe Hospital, a yogurt, ginger biscuits and a brew. Not exactly the fillet steak I had requested but was gratefully received as I was starving.

Have to wait 4 weeks now to make sure that enough nastiness has been removed and that I don't need any further surgery. Then it is radiotherapy.

The staff at Wythenshawe were wonderful and I can't thank them enough for looking after me.

I have had so many cards and gifts it has been unreal but very much appreciated. Beautiful flowers, candles, chocolates, lots of luxurious bath creams, body lotions and tonics, a bookmark, a food box from Dishoom in Manchester to make your own bacon naan flatbreads – a definite recommend. Flower pots for the garden and the list goes on. Oh and not to forget my underarm 'booby cushion' for sleeping which is a god send.

Better still, are the phone calls and messages of support – they are priceless.

Well and truly stuffed

We are truly blessed to have good friends living around us, and more so these last few days after my operation, and whilst we are still both isolating. We were home really late on Thursday and my non FB friends Pat & Mr David (said David☺) had dropped off two pork dinners and her famous yogurt jelly for us, so that was Friday tea sorted. Delicious. Thank you.

Saturday night we were treated to a banging Caribbean curry with all the trimmings from our friends and neighbours 'The Bertellis', Leanne and Mike. Thank you and feel free to share again with us, anytime☺

Sunday we had our roast dinner courtesy of Joe Smith and Lisa Ashworth at our local, The Waggon and Horses. They have been doing takeaways during lockdown. The big man, Joe, delivered ours. Perfect. Thank you

My wonderful friend Sheila tipped up with a veritable feast. A huge pork steak with gorgeous creamy potatoes and red cabbage. Sheila and Phil have not gone without their own struggles with the 'Big C' and are still both here to tell the tale. Amazingly good friends who I love dearly.

Thank you all so much

Much love
Mrs H xx

From my Facebook page – 27 February 2021 – feeling blessed

On a beautiful sunny day we are sitting in the warm sunshine enjoying a gorgeous afternoon tea sent to us by Marjorie – Thank you

We are so grateful for all the gifts I have received and the generosity of friends still feeding us. We have even had Fish and Chip Friday takeaway. A treat indeed.

Our house is bejewelled with flowers and they certainly cheer us up.

Thank you so much

Much love
Mrs H xx

CHAPTER 8
TWO WEEKS POST SURGERY

It has been two weeks since my surgery and I am feeling fine. Yes, it was painful at times but nothing that I could not cope with. I didn't have the luxury of a follow up appointment to make sure that everything was ok and had no follow up with the Consultant either. I basically had a handout from the Hospital showing me what exercises I needed to do to make sure I didn't stiffen up and also to try and avoid getting any lymphedema in my arm.

As the days went by the bruising was like nothing you had ever seen before. I was literally black and blue and every colour in between. It was definitely a Crocodile Dundee moment - 'that's not a bruise, this is a bruise'. Every day there was a change in colour and it was weeks before it lessened to a pasty yellow. I would show you a picture but don't want to put anyone off their tea.

To be quite honest, I was quite worried about the extent of the bruising, and in the absence of any kind of check-up, I spoke to a lovely lady who I know from my time at the Hospice. She was previously a GP, having retired some time ago. The wonderful Dr Elizabeth (Liz) Needham. A pillar of the community. I explained the situation to her and asked if I could pop round for her to have a look. I just needed someone to tell me that things looked ok, that they looked normal. I needed that confirmation to put my mind at rest.

Pop round I did and was treated to some lovely homemade cake and a good cuppa. If you ever saw Liz coming into the Hospice with a cake tin under her arm, you knew you were in for a treat. It was lovely just to talk to someone, a professional. Someone who knew.

It was a bit strange bearing all in her front room I might add, which actually was not at the front, but round the back, but needs must as they say. She gave me a good check over and had a feel around and said that everything looked just fine and as she would have expected at that stage.

Brilliant. I heaved a sigh of relief. She then went on to tell me that she was having trouble with her eyesight and couldn't see very well. Yikes. Now she tells me. We have since spoken about this and had a good laugh. To confirm that day, the tin contained some millionaire shortbread she had made. Perfect.

The Biopsy

I was told that the biopsy would be sent away and that I would have a telephone appointment in about two weeks with- the Consultant.

Nothing much to report about those two weeks. Apart from when you are waiting on a biopsy result, time goes oh so slowly. You count the sleeps, waiting for that day to come. I just rested up the best I could. Watched some Netflix, read, slept and caught up with friends. Mr H was, as usual, a star. Catering to my every whim. Some may say 'what's new' ☺

The day of the phone call arrived, though we were not sure what time it would be. You find yourself constantly looking at the phone, checking it has enough charge, is the volume on and the main thing with me, where actually is my phone as I am a bugger at putting it down and forgetting where it is.

Can't miss that call. It was just a phone call, not even a video call or Skype, of which most of us had become used to. I can remember that when it did ring, my heart felt like it was thumping out of my chest. We both sat at the kitchen table and I had a notebook to hand in case I needed to scribble anything important down. Mr H held onto my hand.

It was Mr Dimopolous, with the Macmillan Nurse,

Nikki, in the background who made the call. Usual pleasantries and then straight to the point. It's good news, no it's great news. The lump is out and the margin that they had taken around it was clear too. That meant no further surgery. The lymph nodes they had removed were also clear.

The feeling of emotion when you are given news like this is indescribable. The relief floods through your veins. You cry when you are given bad news but cry equally as much when you are given good news.

Then there is a BUT, jeez why is there always a BUT!!

It was confirmed that that I had had 'Invasive Ductal Carcinoma' Grade 3 with High Grade Carcinoma in Situ. This is not to be confused with a Stage.

Because of the type of cancer, it was decided that some of my cells would be sent to the USA for some further testing. This test was called an Oncotype DX. What is one of these I hear you ask?

The Oncotype DX is a test that may predict how likely it is that your breast cancer will return. It also predicts whether you will benefit from having chemotherapy in addition to hormone therapy. The test results can help you and your doctors make a treatment plan that's right for you.

The results for this test come back on a scoring

system:

A score between 21 and 25 means you have a medium risk of the cancer returning if you get hormone treatment. The benefits of chemotherapy may outweigh the risk of side effects. A score between 26 and 100 means you have a higher risk that the disease might come back.

Amidst the good news, there was now another cloud hanging over my head. Mr D said that once the results came back, which would probably be another 2 weeks, ahhhh - he would assess and decide whether I should have the Chemotherapy or not.

I had the high of the initial results and then felt like I had been catapulted right back down again.

Life throws us curveballs and this was most certainly one of them, of the highest order. There was not a thing we could do apart from yet another wait. Another two weeks of sleepless nights, counting days, hours, minutes, seconds, because that is what it felt like.

On a lighter note, nobody was able to go away on any exotic holidays, but I can say that part of me flew over that 'Pond' to America ☺ which is further than most folk got.

Wait therefore is what we did. We were advised that

it would be yet another telephone consultation to deliver the next results. It was, therefore the same again. A day of staring at the phone, willing it to ring. We just needed to know.

In brief, the results came back giving me a score of Oncotype 45 – Mr D had discussed my case with other Consultants and they concurred that Chemotherapy was the best option for me. Think of it as belt and braces – it was to make sure. It was an insurance policy.

Mr H was upstairs when this call came through. I climbed the stairs as if my feet were made of lead. This was never in the plan. I had been told at the beginning, that it would be surgery then radiotherapy. I could cope with that. How was I now to deal with this bombshell?

There were tears. Chemo. This is one of those 'C' words that you don't want to hear. Mr H enveloped me in his arms. I was safe there.

He is always very matter of fact, and said that if that is what was needed, so be it. As long as it made me well, we could get through this, together.

I was to be discharged from the Surgical Team at Wythenshawe, and was to be referred to the Oncology Team at the Christie. That 'O' word is another one that I don't like.

CHAPTER 9
MEET THE ONCOLOGIST

My appointment was made to meet the 'Oncologist' a Dr Hannah Chapman. Lucky for me, I was able to see her face to face at the Tameside Macmillan Unit, so no trek over to the 'Mother Ship'.

She was very petite and very young. As long as she knew her stuff, that is all that I cared about. Unfortunately for me, I saw when she stood up that she was rather far into pregnancy and therefore told me that she would not be with me for the whole of my 'journey' – ha, not said it for a while so thought I would slip a quick one in. A Dr Katherine Blake would take over from her when she went on maternity leave.

The appointment was to let me know how the treatment would be given, the timescale and to go through the side effects. I then had to sign to give my consent. She read the full list of side effect to me and I told her that once I got home, the list would be going into a file and it would not see the light of day again.

I will enlighten you with some of those side effects –

of which there were many, but like most drugs, just because there is a side effect on the list, it does not mean that you will get it.

- Tiredness and exhaustion – well Mr H probably won't notice any difference as I can do tired really well already
- Difficulty with concentration and memory – think they call this chemo brain – I will dine out on that one I think
- Tingling, numbness and pain in fingers and toes – known as Peripheral Neuropathy
- Hair loss – this is the main one that I dread
- Weak nails/nail loss – I am not looking forward to the possibility of this one as I have always been fastidious about my nails and caring for them
- Infection
- Death – hang on a minute – not sure about that one, this was supposed to be making me better – she confirmed it was only .1% - ahh so not even a full human
- Nausea & vomiting – I hope not as I hate being sick

Q. Do side effects from chemo get worse with each treatment?
A. The effects of chemo are cumulative. They get worse with each cycle. Each infusion will get harder. With each cycle, expect to feel weaker. Oh Shit!!

I am going to be having two types of chemo. Sarah, my friend, once said that the scientists that make the chemo up are like wizards making magic. I think that this is a good analogy.

Cycle 1 – 3
Epiruicin & Cyclophosphamide

- Given into the vein through a thin tube via a fast-flowing drip. (I have known quite a few drips that have flown through my life rather fast)! I hope more than anything that I have the skills to deal with this particular 'drip' ☺

- Routine blood tests before each treatment – I can deal with that as I have never had a problem parting with blood in the past. Once upon a time I was a regular blood donor. Alas, no more but I have done my bit.

- Immediate effect – giddiness (holy mother of God, will anyone know the difference) – a metallic taste in the mouth – a cold sensation along the course of the vein – dizziness – hair loss

Cycle 4 – 6
Docetaxel (Taxotere)

Most of the side effect are much the same as the first drug, however, there is an extra touch of magic in this drug, but one that means that there is a chance of an allergic reaction, so I was to have the 4th and 5th cycles at the 'Mother Ship' just in case. Better to be safe than sorry. If I had no reactions, I would be able to have the 6th back at Tameside.

- Routine blood tests before each treatment – if the blood count is not at a safe level, the treatment may not go ahead (that's pressure)
- Lethargy – heartburn – joint and muscle pain – changes in nails – sore mouth – skin rash – fluid retention – sensitivity to the sun – strange taste

The more serious ones were:

- Blood clots – hyperpigmentation – infiltration (when chemo leaks outside the vein) – life threatening side effect (none listed for this but SHIT)!! Don't care now, I've said it

So there I had it, I was in possession of the full facts and just needed to sign on the dotted line. Of which obviously I did.

She told me there and then when I would be starting and of all the dates in the whole 365 days of the year, I was to have my first Cycle on the 7 May, my birthday. Happy Birthday to me.

Que Sera Sera (Whatever will be)

This was going to be a journey like no other – I must tread carefully and listen to my body. I must realise the importance of taking small steps and not try to run before I can walk.

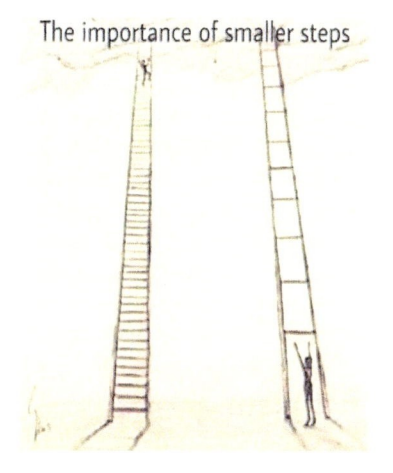

The importance of smaller steps

CHAPTER 10
LET'S GET WIGGY WITH IT

I had many a conversation with my 'Oracles', Sarah and Caroline – I called them my Martini Girls as they had both said that I could ring them literally, 'Any time, any place, anywhere'.

I was under no illusion that I would lose my hair. They both had, so why would I be any different. I wanted to make sure that I had all my ducks in line before I started, as I was not sure how I would be after the first chemo and whether I would be well enough to go shopping for the 'essentials' that I would need.

I had also spoken to them both about the benefits of wearing the 'cold cap'.

Q. Do cold caps work with chemo?
A. Cold caps and scalp cooling systems work by narrowing the blood vessels beneath the skin of the scalp, which reduces the amount of chemotherapy medicine that reaches the hair follicles. With less chemotherapy medicine in the follicles, the hair may be less likely to fall out.

They both had tried wearing one only once. They add hours onto your treatment, as you need to wear them for about an hour before and then an hour after and the gunk they have to put on your hair is enough to make it fall out anyway.

Sarah said that it was excruciatingly cold and painful and that it gave her the mother of all headaches, and Caroline said that during the time she had it on, it was as if she was having some kind of funny turn and could not get her words out so they had to whip it off.

My hairdresser had done lots of research and her findings were that the extreme cold would stress the hair follicles every time and that if, and it was always going to be an if, you managed to keep hold of any hair, it would be in a terrible condition.

Armed with all this information, I made the decision that I would not be going down this route. I love a hat, don't get me wrong, the bigger the better, and they are usually extremely stylish and large.

If you ever find yourself or someone you know in this position, I made this decision after lots of research and speaking to other people, but we are all different and what is right for one person is not always right for another.

Jeremy No 1

Wigs it was then, or as I like to call them a 'Jeremy Jigg'. As we were still in lockdown, I had to make an appointment at a shop in Manchester – Salon Maier, and they would only allow me in the shop for the appointment. I had spent hours trawling through their brochure online and had in mind what I thought would suit me.

The day of the appointment met us with glorious sunshine. Mr H obviously took me down to Manchester, dropping me off right outside the shop and then went to park up.

The young girl in the shop was lovely and put me at ease straight away. The shop has been there for many years and has a good reputation so they knew what they were doing. This was before I started my treatment so I still had my own hair, though I can't remember if I had already had it cut short at this stage. I showed her the kind of styles I quite liked and she set about finding the ones I wanted to try on. Damn COVID – she had quite a few of the styles I liked but not in the colour I needed, and their policy at that time was that they could be tried on only once and then had to go into quarantine.

Note to self: never dye my hair black or ginger (or anything on that spectrum of colour). I looked like something out of a horror show.

I decided that I liked the Raquel Welch wigs the best, as most of them had roots and looked very natural and real. I learned that a lace front was best, as if I wanted I could clip the front back and could change which side I wanted the parting to go. Wow, this sounds easier than dealing with your own hair.

I finally decided on a just off the shoulder, ash blonde, wavy, rooted, lace front one. I had been sending Mr H photos for his approval and we both liked the same one best. By the time I had had numerous wigs on and off, my hair was plastered down to my head. Oh no, as the weather was so nice, we had decided to stay in Manchester for some lunch.

I had no option, 'Jeremy' was going to have to make its debut appearance. I won't lie, it wasn't cheap – probably the equivalent of say 4 visits to Tony & Guy, but to me it was worth every penny. I have always taken pride in my appearance and done many creative things with my hair. If I was to feel comfortable and not in that 'comfy' way, I mean in how I looked, then it had to be right. Purchase duly made and off I trotted to meet Mr H.

It felt strange at first, especially when I caught sight of myself in the shop windows. It was a complete change. A different colour, much shorter length, no fringe and not as much height as I usually like on top.

Shock, horror!! I decided to walk through Kendals – now that is really showing my age as it has been House of Fraser for years. I was going to be ok. Nobody was staring at me. Nobody knew. This was to be the new me, for a while at least. I better make a purchase ☺ well it would be rude not to.

I found Mr H and we decided as it was such a nice day that we would have our lunch out in the sunshine in St Ann's Square. Though really sunny, there was quite a wind whipping down from the side streets. Yikes, this was going to be a test. Would Jeremy stay put, would he cut the mustard? I can confirm that Jeremy 1 sufficiently passed the wind tunnel test, in fact with flying colours.

Jeremy No 2

What I have not told you yet is that you get a voucher to spend on wigs from the NHS, but typical for me, you could not redeem it at the shop I got Jeremy 1 from.

I decided that I might as well see what they had to offer with my NHS voucher and headed off to what was actually a unit situation on a Stockport Business Park. Again, another lovely lady who could not do enough to help. Thinking about it, I must still have had my long hair as it was clipped up at the back and I explained that I rarely had my hair down and that I doubted she would be able to sort me out with anything similar to my own.

Wrong – she brought out a long wig with a fringe, almost the same colour as my own hair. She put it on me, got my clip and just like that it looked like me. Wowzer. Amazing. She just needed to trim the fringe slightly and honestly, you would not know. So now we have 'Jeremy 2'. Months down the line, I would call into my hairdresser and Gemma would do some creative plaiting and messy style buns. It really did look like me.

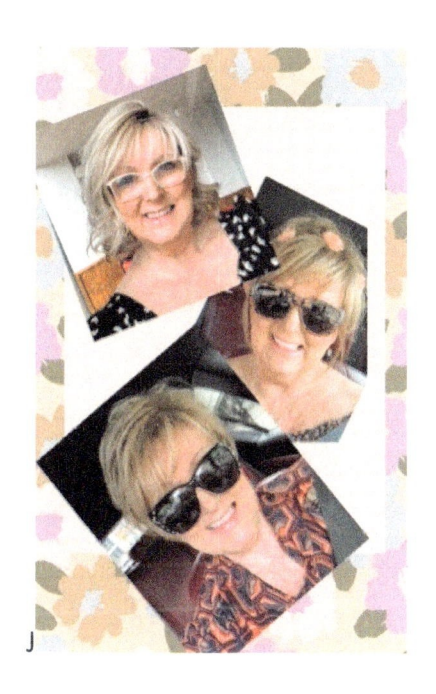

Jeremy 1,2 & 3

Jeremy 3

When my hair eventually started growing, I decided to invest in 'Jeremy 3'. I know, greedy. It's the future. Let's face it, many pop stars and big movie stars wear them all the time and nobody blinks an eye. If it's good enough for them, it's good enough for me.

Back to Salon Maier. I wanted a shorter more cropped style to try and ease me gently into having short hair. Raquel Welch to the rescue again and yet another lace front, rooted specimen. Jeremy 1 was my first love but Jeremy 3 is the one that most people liked the most.

So that you will be pleased to know is wig shopping over and done with.

What I have not mentioned yet, is that the hair disappears from everywhere and I mean everywhere.

I had again anticipated beforehand that my eyebrows would be disappearing and took the plunge to have them microbladed. Bearing in mind that I don't like pain, I was slightly worried about this and in fact felt more anxious than when I had the surgery. I was also stressed that I would come out looking like I had a couple of slugs crawling across my forehead!

I need not have worried. I can't say that it didn't hurt but it was bearable. The weirdest thing was that the implement they use felt like it was scratching through to my skull.

If you don't know what microblading is, then just imagine someone cutting tiny nicks into your eyebrows with a razor blade like implement and then dropping ink into the cuts! So in effect, tattooing your skin. Wow, mad.

I am so glad that I made this decision as when the eyebrows eventually disappeared, I still had a frame to my face. To me this was important to try and keep some of my identity.

Let us now address nostril hair. Yuk. But we all have it. It's just there doing what it does, but have you ever thought what that is? I love a good Google so this is what it says.

Nose hair is an important part of your body's defense system. It helps keep dust, allergens, and other small particles from entering your lungs. Removing too much hair may make you more sensitive to these kinds of debris. Plucking your hairs can also lead to irritation, infections, and ingrown hairs

Can't say that I noticed any debris flying around my snout, but it ran like a flippin tap. Very annoying, so it is a good job that I had that stash of hankies down my cleavage☺

There has to be some good in everything and I was happy to take whatever that good happened to be. Shall we just call it 'body hair loss'. Yehh smooth, hair free legs. Now that was a bonus. I don't need to go any further about this fact but just to say that when it starts to come back, it's bloody itchy☺

CHAPTER 11
FEELING BLESSED

From my Facebook page – 6 May 2021 – feeling blessed

Dear friends, it is some time since I have done one of my epic posts, so strap yourself in, get a brew and a biscuit and here we go.

It is my birthday tomorrow. Just an ordinary birthday, not a milestone one or anything like that. I have broken with tradition today as I never open cards or presents beforehand, but this year is different. To say that I am overwhelmed with the cards, gifts and flowers is somewhat of an understatement.

You see tomorrow is going to be a birthday like no other. You see it is the first day of, to quote that cliché again 'the next part of my journey'. The first day of my chemotherapy.

My actual surgery was a success and they got rid of everything they needed to, but on the back of some further testing in America, it was decided that it would be beneficial for me to have the chemo to lessen the chance of any recurrence in the future. So that is what is happening. 6 rounds in 3 week cycles. Not the best birthday present, but in a way it is.

Since I started on this 'journey' oh no, I have said it again. I have had two other friends who have joined me in this 'exclusive club'. So once again, I reiterate even more the importance of getting yourself checked if you are in any doubt.

If something does not feel right, do not leave it to chance.

Chemo Day – My Birthday - Tumour Humour Alert

They say "laughter is the best medicine" – unless you have cancer, then chemotherapy is more effective ☺

My dilemma is 'what do I take with me'? Their response was to pack things you would take in say a flight bag. Oh no! Those who have ever travelled with me know that I do not pack lightly. In fact, if I do not get a heavy sticker on at least one of my bags, I feel like I have done myself an injustice. Think I may have already mentioned that so claiming 'chemo brain'. I may just draw the line at taking my 4-way extending extension reel. I kid you not, I have been caught out too many times on holiday, with the mirror being on one side of the room and the plug socket on the other. Mr H has on numerous occasions had to move mirrors and light fittings.

What shall I wear? Maybe a tracksuit they said or dare I say it 'something comfy' ahhhh! Firstly, do I look like an athlete? Secondly, that particular 'C' word is not in my vocabulary.

Mr H and I want to thank everyone for the continued kindness and care shown to us. We have an amazing support network and that means so much to us.

I want to thank my 'Human Breast Cancer Wikipedia Friends' – Caroline, Sarah, Daniella, Nicky & Naz. We have all walked in the same shoes. I thank them for their support, guidance and knowledge from having been there.

So 'Hold that Crown' for me for a while as I will be back in the not too distant future and it will be back firmly in place.

Much love
Mrs H xx

When someone you love has a cancer diagnosis, it's hard to know what to do or what to say. Thoughtful and sincere sympathy messages are wonderful. But to be quite honest, we sometimes grow tired of earnest displays of emotion. The sideways sympathy glance. The look of pity. Just because someone is sick, it doesn't mean they lose their sense of humour. I certainly didn't. That makes me sound ungrateful, and believe me – I am 100% not. I cherished every phone call and message. I just didn't want to admit that I was ill and in some ways be treated as such.

If you are ever in the position with a loved one, just be yourself - just be normal. Some normality in this pantomime is good.

I think it shocked some people in that I was not displaying the typical cancer/chemo patient traits. I didn't want to think of myself as being ill. Yes, I had the blasted thing, but after surgery, I was simply having treatment. Yes, sometimes I did not quite feel myself, and I had the side effects to prove it, but I didn't want to be that person who played the sympathy card. It was my way of coping.

I was lucky.

CHAPTER 12
CHEMOTHERAPY

Here's some science for you.

Q. How does chemotherapy work?

A. It is a drug that targets cells that grow and divide quickly, as cancer cells do. Unlike radiation or surgery, which target specific areas, chemo can work throughout your body. But it can also affect some fast-growing healthy cells, like those of the skin, hair, intestines, and bone marrow.

I become quite an expert in all things cancer/chemo related and that is something I never thought I would be saying.

I had the dates for my treatments and they refer to them as 'Cycles' and not the ones with wheels on. I was to have 6 Cycles, 1 every third week and mine were to be on a Friday.

When you are told that you need chemo, all kinds of things go through your head as historically we heard so many bad things about it, with patients being really sick and more. I had no idea how I would handle it. How it would affect me. I spoke to my 'Warrior' friends and they told me about the extreme tiredness, the nausea, hair loss and much more.

We are of course all different, and I could only hope that I was strong enough to deal with whatever cards I was to be dealt. My main worry was losing my hair. My crown and glory. The nurse told me that it would happen and that I should perhaps prepare beforehand and get my hair cut shorter, to kind of get used to when it fell out. I can tell you, 100% and most categorically, that nothing, not one thing can prepare you for when that happens.

I had to face the fact so I did as suggested and my lovely hairdresser, Gemma, said she would come and cut it for me.

I had always wanted long hair when I was a child, but it never seemed to go further than my shoulders. I wanted to be like my cousins, Sue, Sheila, Lesley, Christine, Pat and Joyce. They all had the Middlehurst 'long hair' gene. It is only in the last few years that I have actually managed to cultivate such locks, though strangely enough, I almost never wear it down as it 'gets on my nerves'. Try then to imagine how I felt, how you would feel, knowing that it would soon be gone.

Gemma had been an absolute star, coming every Friday to blow my hair as I couldn't hold the hairdryer up for any length of time. Mr H had bought me a Dyson hairdryer just before all the shenanigans began. Thinking back, I should have put it out for rent as I would not be requiring its services for quite some time. My hair was that thick, I could put it in a wet bun in the morning and it still be damp at the end of the day.

On the day she came to cut it short, I sat there staring into the mirror, trying to be brave but failing miserably. She put it into two ponytails and then 'snip, snip' it was all gone. I sobbed like a baby as she handed them to me, safely encased in elastic bands. I still have them on my dressing table and often hold them to my face, breathing in the smell of the shampoo that still lingers.

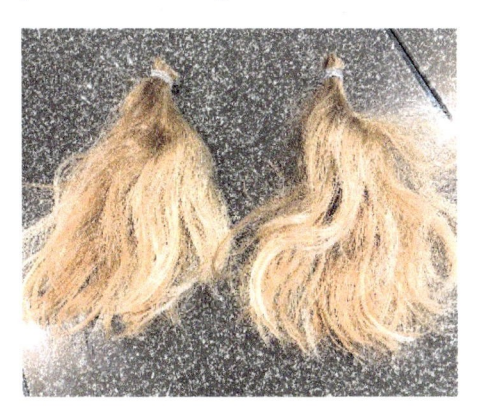

She cut it high into the nape of my neck but left me some length at the front as I was due to go to my friend's wedding and still hoped that it would stay long enough for me to have some sort of style.

Thankfully it did, just.

CHAPTER 13
SCARED OF STALYBRIDGE BUT ACTUALLY TERRIFIED OF TAMESIDE

CHEMOTHERAPY – 6 x Rounds – 1 every 3 weeks

Whilst you have been reading this you may think that I have been quite blasé about things. I know I try to put a humorous spin on events but I am telling you now, that I was scared. I was petrified of having this chemo. We have all seen the images on TV, adverts for Macmillan, pictures in a magazine. People looking poorly. How could this be me? I had no idea of how I was going to react to the treatment. People say to keep positive and for most of the time, I do try. If you are going to have a hard time with it, positivity cannot help with the medical facts. It can however help you with your wellbeing and mind-set. Mr H has drummed this in to me for years.

I think I have touched on this subject slightly before, in that I am a really closed book. I do not like people seeing me upset, stressed or anxious. I am a good actress. I feel that if I display these traits, that I have failed myself. That I am weak. I now know that this is a ridiculous thing to think of myself. Only Mr H knows. I rarely confide in anyone. I am a very private person. Maybe this is not good, but it is who I am and I am a bit long in the tooth for this behaviour to change now. If I do not share my feelings with you, don't be offended. It is nothing you have done.

I hoped with all my being that I would be fine with the treatment. It was again like going into the unknown, into the lion's den. I literally was David and if felt like the chemo was Goliath. But, I am strong. I am not weak and I was determined I would do my best to deal with whatever was thrown at me.

I know some people have a really tough time with their treatments and my heart goes out to those who suffer. We have all heard horror stories of someone we know, a friend of a friend, so and so next door who had an absolute torturous time.

I know that this is going to be tough but hopefully, please, let it not be too bad for me. I will do a forfeit afterwards – promise - anything.

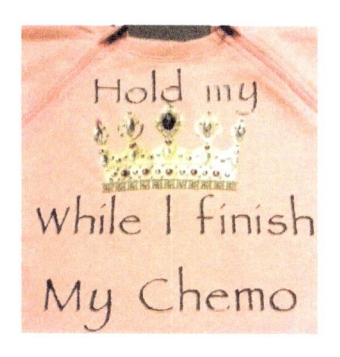

This was my chemo plan. Not much when you say it quick, but when you add it all up, it is the best part of 18 weeks, almost 4 months. How spooky that it was to start on my birthday and end on Chris's.

I was lucky. In Tameside, there is a Macmillan Unit with a small Chemo Suite. There are 6 chairs set in a semi-circle and they look out onto a lovely courtyard. The nurses from The Christie come to this Unit to administer the drugs. I was to have the first 3 rounds there, then two at The Christie, or the 'Mother Ship' as I like to call it, and then the last one back at Tameside.

The 4th and 5th cycles needed to be given at The Christie, as with this change of drug, there was a slight change of having some kind of allergic reaction. They wanted you there as they have more staff on hand if there are any problems.

I had been in constant discussion with my two 'Oracles', Sarah and Caroline. I wanted to know how it had been for them. I wanted it warts and all.

Caroline took the more softer approach, and whilst not holding anything back told me how it had been for her. Her biggest advice was that I should 'PACE' myself. Listen to my body and if it wanted to rest, then rest it must. She said to watch myself with the munchies as she had been up on many a long night, scoffing on 'Crunchy Nut Cornflakes – other products are however available.

Sarah's rendition was much more gritty and graphic and I would not have expected anything else from her. She had had a much tougher experience and as a Police Office with many years' service and having experienced things we can only imagine, she had a much harder time. 'PACE' for Sarah however meant a completely different thing (you would have to be in 'The Job') to understand that one – google it.

Unfortunately, Sarah was one of the unlucky ones who had an allergic reaction to the 4th Cycle. That my friends, is why they wanted you at the 'Mother Ship'. The staff were around her like bees round honey. It must have been very scary for her but they managed the situation like the professionals they are, and she was fine. Thank God.

Caroline donned the wig and Sarah didn't as she could not get along with it. When I told her how much I had paid for mine, she thought that perhaps the £60 she had parted with may have had something to do with it.

I have had a conversation with Sarah and she says that if by any chance my book is made into a film ☺ can Angeline Jolie play her. I asked Mr H who should play me? His response without hesitation was Charlize Theron – ohh secret crush me thinks. He does not deny this saying that she is a 'bit nice'. Caroline says that in her dreams, Courtney Cox will be tipping up to play her. So that's that sorted.

CHAPTER 14
CHEMO 1, FIRST CYCLE – 7 MAY 2021

As I have said previously, it was my birthday. My 58th birthday. Not one I would forget in a hurry. I had had a lovely day the day before, albeit that I had to go and get my bloods done. Friends had called around and it was like no other birthday. The presents, cards and flowers were just everywhere, on every available surface. Overwhelmingly generous gifts. It freaked me slightly. Were these extraordinary gestures of kindness because they thought it would be my last birthday? Stupid I know, but these are the kind of thoughts that go rushing round your head, tormenting and torturing. Mr H as usual, put short shrift to that though, telling me not to be so daft, of course it wouldn't be my last!! The day had been a mixture of emotions and gratitude and the amount of love and support around me was truly amazing.

The first 'Cycle' was at the Macmillan Unit in Tameside, that luckily for us, is literally 10 minutes down the road. I had packed my bag the night before. A new rucksack – Steve Madden don't you know – I had never had a rucksack before, not really having needed one. I love my bags as like shoes, you can always rely on them fitting you. On this occasion, it was perfect and did the job nicely.

I was loaded up with iPad, iPhone, charger, book, toffees, slippers, blanket, lip salve, notebook and lots more. As I was not sure what the facilities were, I also took along a flask of coffee, a flask of Vimto and my own cup. I looked like I was going for the weekend not just a few hours. Standard behaviour from Mrs H.

Mr H dropped me at the door. Others had offered to take me but Mr H would not hear of it. I have said before, he would take me to the ends of the earth and beyond if he could.

I sat in the waiting room that was actually a big kitchen but with soft furnishings and magazines. The wait is always the worst I think as you are stepping into boundaries that you know nothing about. Thankfully, the wait was not too long.

A Health Care Assistant who I now know as Aidee, came to collect me. A big lad – I don't mean BIG, but tall and a with a presence if you know what I mean. He had a huge bushy beard sticking out from his mask and a Phil Mitchell style head, if you know what I mean. Now he definitely had lovely eyes. Piercing blue and oozing care and love. I will tell you more about Aidee later, but we became good friends.

I was taken to my chair, note not a bed, which I think is good. A bed seems so much more clinical. There were only two other patients having treatment that day so it felt really friendly and intimate. First things first and Aidee did the brew run. At first I said no as I had taken my own, but then I decided to have one of theirs. My lovely coffee cup from John Lewis was produced as I said to Aidee that I didn't like drinks out of paper cups. His response 'Ohh we've got a Princess here'. We were going to get on just fine.

It was a good brew too. The brews there were always good, and always accompanied with a plate of some kind of goodies. Well it would be rude not to, so I always accepted what was offered.

THE GOODY BAG

It seemed like there was always something on offer whilst I sat in my chariot. This time Aidee was giving out 'Goody Bags' that had been donated by a local charity. Mossley Cancer Committee to be precise. My first instinct was to decline. Why would I need such a thing? I was lucky in that I had everything that I could possibly want and more. I did, however, have a re-think and decided to accept said bag with the grace in which it had been given. I was so glad that I did.

The bag contained lots of lovely things that would help you hopefully feel that little bit better. Lip-gloss, boiled sweets, paper hankies, pens, puzzle books, hand cream and much more. How amazing. I will touch on this more in Chemo 3.

I always thought, well that is not quite true as I suppose it is not really something you think about, but I must have seen pictures, that they hooked you up to your chemo drip and left you to it. I was surprised, therefore when my nurse pulled up her chair and wheeled her trolley over, bit like being on a BA flight but without the G&T or duty-free goods☺ In reality, what was contained on that trolley was so much more than a warmish glass of prosecco and a tub of Pringles. It was the 'magic' trolley.

My nurse was Thea. I have said this about all the professionals that looked after me, but she really was wonderful. We had some lovely conversations. Normal conversations. She explained that for this particular drug, she would sit with me, making sure that it did not seep into the wrong veins. Not all nurses have the training to give this particular drug, so it was proper 'technical' stuff going on. It was quite high-tech really, with all the information she needed on a laptop that moved everywhere with her.

I had set my stall out on the table at the side of my chair, bringing with me one birthday card, obviously the one from Mr H, a bendy flower attached to the arm of my chair, my coffee flask, cup and a couple of biscuits. As it was a really hot day, I also had a glass bottle with a cold drink. Well, would you believe it, the chemo was the exact same colour as my Vimto.

The syringes sat there on 'that trolley' and for all the world it looked like she was going to shove my drink of choice into my veins.

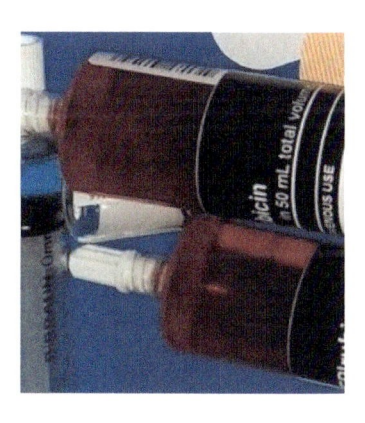

To start with, she flushed some kind of saline through before starting with the chemo. I have 'really good' veins apparently. Nice and fat and squishy. Perfect for that cannula. So there it was, Chemo No 1 on its way. I didn't really know what to expect. For me, it was quite uneventful. I felt a slight coldness searing through but apart from that not much else. I had no idea how long it would take as again, you hear of some folk who have chemo taking hours. I was, therefore, pleasantly surprised to be told that as mine was going through really well, it would only take just over an hour. Flippin eck. Mr H would just be getting home and would have to come back to get me.

At the end of the actual chemo going in there was another solution put through. I was told that I may experience a slight tingling sensation in my nose. Weird. Well, I must be a textbook patient as almost as soon as it went in, my nose started to tingle. Oh no. I could feel a sneeze building up. If you have ever been in my company when I sneeze, then you will know that firstly there is rarely a single sneeze and secondly, that if you were recording the decibels, I would score quite highly. I used to work in an open plan office and at almost the same time every day I would start to sneeze, no idea why. There was a 'behind locked doors' office next to where I sat and they would knock on the wall and tell me to 'shut up'. That's how loud I am☺

So there it was, I started to sneeze. Probably a good ten, rip roaring sneezes. I apologised profusely to my fellow patients in between every one and to be quite honest, I got on my own nerves. Cleavage hankies to the rescue.

Chemo 1 done and dusted and Mr H was summoned to come and collect me. I was provided with a bag full of drugs, the main players being a set of syringes that I was informed needed to be stuck in my belly for the next 7 days. Chemo whilst killing bad cells, also does the same to good cells so these injections were to build my immune system back up. One of the biggest risk is infection as chemo affects your immune system. It affects the white blood cells so these injections were very important.

I don't know what I expected to feel once I got home. I had just had chemo so I thought I would need to take to my bed - that I would feel poorly. Bed, therefore is where I went. Not in bed you understand, but propped up with a brew, my cats and the TV.

It was weird. I felt ok. That was good but it was not what I thought I would feel like. I am not sure if it was my imagination but I just felt a bit weird. Not quite myself. Nothing major though. Nothing I could put my finger on. I could smell something strange. But could I? Was it my imagination! It wasn't a bad smell, just one I had not smelt before. It might have just been the enormity of the day, making that brain play tricks on me again.

You hear about 'the sickness' that comes with chemo and that is one thing that I dreaded. I was armed with anti-sickness tablets and my 'Oracles' had told me not to wait until I felt sick, but to take them 3 times a day as prevention. Prevention as they say is better than cure. That is what I did. I was again lucky I think, as I was not sick even once throughout the whole of the treatment cycles.

Nothing much to report for the rest of that night really. There were lots of phone calls and messages checking in to see how I was. I was ok.

For the next 7 days, I was to have the injections that they had given me. Mr H put them in a butty box in the fridge. Very medical that. I am quite a tough cookie but I cannot even pull a plaster off without screaming like a piglet. There was no way I could administer those injections myself. Mr H would have to step up to the mark. Step up he did. A right little Dr Kildare. Mask on, rubber gloves on, syringe at the ready. Pinch the inch they said ☺ that was not going to be a problem. I need not have worried, as the injections were painless. We decided to do them on opposite sides each day so as not to have me ending up looking like a pincushion.

Day 1 – 6 no problem at all. Day 7 started off ok, but as the day went on I ended up with the mother of all backaches. Pains that sent spasms up my back giving me the shakes. It lasted for hours. It was a hot day but I needed a hot water bottle to try and ease the pain. These days were the only time I took to my bed. Wrapped up tight in the duvet. We subsequently worked out that this was something that happened on the 7th day every time. It was not nice, but if this was a bad as it was to get, I was ok with it. I just had to grin and bear it and rest up the best I could.

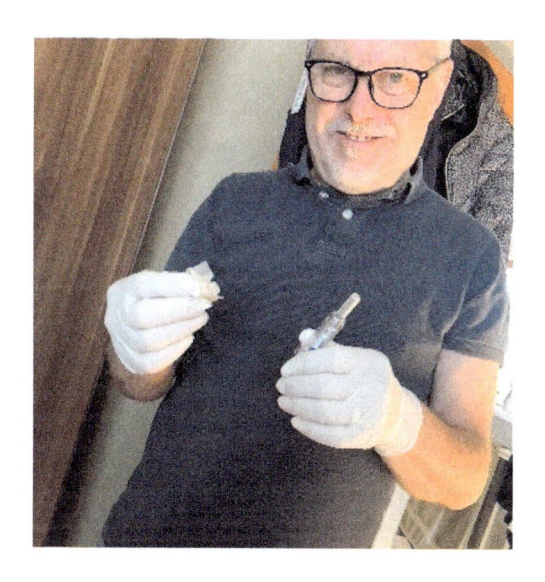

'Sometimes the thing we need most, is to give ourselves permission to rest'

There was nothing much to report really for the next 3 weeks. As I write this, I realise that this is actually a big fat lie.

I had been to my friend's wedding and my hair was just about hanging on. I still managed the style I wanted with my new shorter bob and my beautiful fascinator.

It was about 2 ½ weeks in that the worst thing ever happened. The thing that I had been dreading the most. I know I sound superficial and vain. I did not want that to be the case but you will agree that hair is part of your image, the way the world sees you when you step outside. I have always taken great care with my hair, wearing in all kinds of styles. All I could think about was what would I look like? I was prepared - but not prepared. Friends would tell me that it did not matter, that I was still me. It did matter. It mattered to me.

I had noticed that when I ran my hands through my hair, it was coming out in clumps. It needed washing but I was frightened to death of doing it. It had not however been coming out on my pillow during the night. At least I did not wake up every morning to that vision.

I had to take the plunge and wash it. I have never felt as anxious. I massaged the shampoo in with feather like touches. So far so good. I dabbed it dry, not wanted to stress any of the follicles that had actually started to hurt, you know like when you have had a tight bobble in for too long. I had to use the hairdryer though, as I have never had the kind of hair that you can just 'wash and go'. I hope my dear friend, known as RBH (Ruth Bradley-Holt) will have a read of this book and laugh when she sees this. 'Wash and go' is one of her many catchphrases.

Mr H knew how stressed I was. We had talked briefly about what we would do when the time came and we both knew that it was almost upon us. I aimed the dryer at my head from a distance to try and take the dampness out. Mr H was side on to me in his office working and I did not know that he was looking. But looking he was and he came to tell me that just the force of the dryer was too much. The hair was flying out at the back of me. There were tears in his eyes. There were now clumps of baldness at the sides. I would never go out with it looking like it did.

It was time.

We had decided that Mr H would use his clippers. We both sat on the floor. He started. We were both crying, sobbing. This should not be happening to me. As I type this, months down the line when my hair is growing back well, I have to stop as the tears are falling down my face. My eyes are blurred and I cannot see the screen.

The sobbing continued. I looked at myself in the mirror. I was no Sinead O'Connor for sure. How people actually do this for charity is beyond me, though I know they do it for good reasons.

I wanted to be on my own. Just for a short while to collect my thoughts. It was a strange feeling actually, but I eventually calmed down. The worst had happened now. I no longer had to stress about it. The fear of the loss had now gone. I needed to pull my big girl knickers up and try to get on with it. Easier said than done, but I gave it my best shot and think I did ok.

I eventually let Mr H back in the room. It was a glorious day. He told me to get my slap on, put my wig on as we were going out. And that, is what we did. There was never any question that I would go wig free. I am not that brave. I have friends who have done this and I take my hat off to them, but not my wig ☺

Jeremy 1 made his second appearance. I felt ok. Like the first time when I had just bought it, nobody stared. Nobody knew. I was going to be all right.

NO MATTER HOW YOU FEEL
GET UP, DRESS UP, SHOW UP
AND NEVER
GIVE UP
(Regina Brett)

Backtracking slightly, it was months after that my dear friend, Aunty Jean (as you know, she is not my real Aunty but almost the real thing), told me that in those first few weeks when I called on her, she recalled that on one occasion I had a navy sweatshirt on. I remember the one. What I did not know is that when I got up to go, I left a raft of hair on the back of the couch. She had to get the hoover out and she too sobbed.

The rest of the time before the next cycle passed without much to report. I sat out in the garden with my sunhat on under my brolly, as you have to be careful not to get sun burnt. I am not much of a sun worshiper anyway, so if you see me with any kind of tan, it is most likely out of a bottle. I had bought a couple of really large 'film star' like sunhats, and wore them usually with a silky scarf underneath, with a fashionably tied knot at the side.

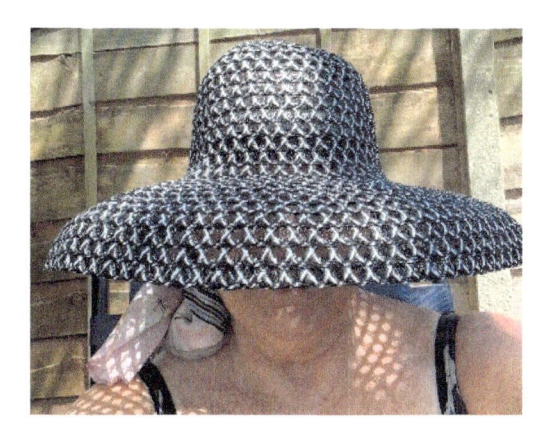

Here we go off on a tangent again☺ I am a fan of the ripped jean and if I am wearing them I put false tan only on the bits where the holes are. Waste not want not. I have told Mr H that if I ever have an accident and need to go to hospital, if they have to remove my jeans he must tell them that I do not have some kind of deadly skin disease, but that it is just my false tan blotched here and there).

CHAPTER 15
CHEMO CYCLES 2 & 3

Chemo 2 – Second Cycle – 28 May 2021

This second cycle came around really quite quickly. It may be because mine were on a Friday but week 2 came around almost immediately and then the third was already in sight. I was more prepared this time, toning down the amount of paraphernalia I took with me. I did however take my own cup with me again, though this time the John Lewis one was substituted with my 'Joanne, Queen of Stalybridge' mug. Aidee thought this hilarious, laughing that I had been promoted to a Queen, from a Princess.

The actual treatment was the same as the first one, with the same bag of tablets and syringes handed to me at the end.

It is funny how you forget some of the finer details, but I think I was given some steroids to take. I must have been, as I was worried that they would give me what I call 'moon face' but was told that I was not going to be on them long enough. Phew that was all I needed.

I had the 7 x days of injections again and the same thing happened on the 7th day, with the back spasms and pain. At least I was expecting it this time. Still no sickness and I still felt well. I hoped with all hope that this would continue.

From my Facebook page – 5 June 2021 – feeling perplexed – somewhere in the middle of the night

For those of you who know my sleeping habits, the middle of the night is a time that I have not witnessed since those days back in my 20s and 30s, slipping home with the milkman (not literally) from Carriages, Cherries or Bredbury Hall (all nightclubs in the Manchester area). Dodgy place Bredbury Hall☺ not really as I met Mr H there.

I had a bad day yesterday with mega pains in my back and it took hours to get that under control. On a hot day like it was, I was wrapped in my duvet with a heat pad trying to make the pain stop.

Good news, it has almost gone so Saturday is a new day and one nearer the finishing line.

No alternative but to get my book out and have a good laugh (reading Romesh Ranganathan's, As Good as It Gets). I am not on any kind of commission, but it's a recommend from me.

Happy middle of the night

Much Love
Mrs H xx

Chemo 3 – Third Cycle – 18 June 2021

Still at the Macmillan Unit at Tameside and I am now getting used to the procedures and the set up. I did not feel the anxiety and stress when being dropped off and in fact, felt quite blasé about the whole thing. Off I trotted into the Unit, barely giving a backwards glance.

I had to go the day before to have bloods done, as if there are any problems, you cannot have your treatment. It was great being able to go to the Tameside Unit as there literally was no waiting time. I even cheekily parked in the drop off area outside. Well, I was dropping my blood off☺

It was really comforting as well, that most of the time it was the same staff. It is about the only time during the whole experience that I was able to make any real connections with anyone. As a community, it is brilliant that we have this facility right on our doorstep and for me, it took away the pressure of the travelling and waiting at 'The Mother Ship'.

Aidee, the Health Care Assistant was there and as usual, greeted me like a long lost friend. My mug of choice this time had progressed again, from Queen, to Duchess. This always made him laugh. Heaven know what he must have thought of me. I may give off vibes of poshness and most certainly play up to this title, but in reality, I am actually 'Mrs Down to Earth from Droylsden'. Just for the record, I do like a nice mug and have quite a large collection that drives Mr H to distraction, especially when trying to balance them on top of each other in the cupboard!

The treatment cycle again went as planned and was much the same as the first two. I was asked how my feet were, which at the time I thought a very strange question! I will cover why this was a recurring question later in Chemo 5.

Mr Banks

I had also made friends with David Banks who is the Manager of the Unit and it was on this visit, that he asked could he interview me for one of the local rags. This was about the fundraising I had done for Mossley Cancer Committee. Remember, the chemo bags.

Interview completed and photo duly taken. I emphasised that it might have been my idea in the first place, but an idea is only an idea and the thanks really went to all my friends for their generosity in donating because without them it would have been just that, an idea.

No Paparazzi

How exciting, I have made one of the local rags, even though they spelt my name wrong, but if you know me, you know me. The article was a little about me, but mainly about the fundraising.

Mr H goes on about people spelling our name wrong, and he has had to put up with this much longer than me. How hard is to get 5 letters in the correct order? He once told me of an occasion when he worked for a Japanese Company and they had 5 of the top Management over visiting. There was a welcome board in the reception with all the names on and the only one spelt wrong was Hinds!! Not Furakawa, Takashima, Suzuki or Kasaki – just ours, one of the all-time favourites, Hines.

The chemo bags I mentioned handed to me at Chemo 1, certainly had lots of lovely things in them to make your life a little bit easier and comfortable. This gave me the idea to give something back to the charity that had so thoughtfully donated these. I canvassed my friends and family for donations to give to the charity so they could buy things to put into the bags.

I was inundated with either lovely thoughtful items or money to buy things. Everyone was so kind and generous. Mr H and I went shopping and we filled a whole trolley with goodies. We had so much stuff that when I delivered it to the lady who is involved in the charity, the lovely Valerie Lee, who I now call one of my dear friends, I had to put the seats down in the back of the car to fit it all in. She was over the moon. This was going to make a difference to so many people.

Oh, the excitement of seeing yourself in print. Copies of the paper were bought and duly given out to anyone who wanted one, and to those who didn't! It really made me laugh about the incorrect spelling of 'Hinds'. It is only 5 little letters, but you would not believe how many different ways we see it spelt. It still felt surreal to see myself sat in that chemo chair.

That was never supposed to be me ☹

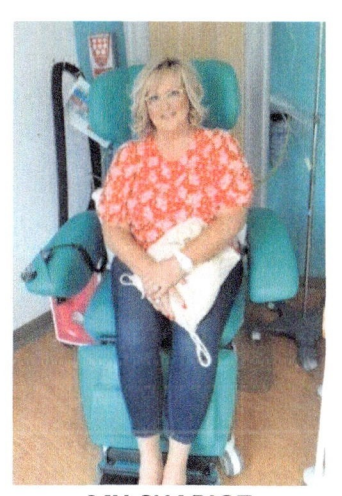

MY CHARIOT

Cycles 1,2 & 3 done and dusted.

CHAPTER 16
CHEMO 4 & 5 @ THE 'MOTHER SHIP'

Chemo 4 – Fourth Cycle – 9 July 2021

This was to be my first encounter at the 'Mother Ship'. It is about a 20 mile round trip journey for us. Not too bad, but if the appointment was anywhere near rush hour, it became an actual nightmare of a journey. It was going to be a totally different experience. I had to go the day before my treatment for my bloods to be taken, which was a bit of a pain, not literally though, as it did not hurt☺ but you know what I mean.

I had to queue up outside the actual building, and the queue I might add was usually quite lengthy. Masks on and as you entered they fired a thermometer at your head, asking you various questions about your visit and checking that you had no VID symptoms. Still nobody else allowed in with me, so I had to go it alone once again.

At least they had a M&S Café there so I was guaranteed a good cup of coffee.

I parked myself in the waiting room and waited – and waited. They have big screens that flash up with your name when it is your turn. I tried to read my book but kept reading the same bit over again as I was constantly checking the screen.

It was so busy there. Just in that waiting room, there must have been 50 or more patients. Some for bloods and some waiting to be called up to the chemo suite. Not at all what I had become used to.

I was back to the insistent waiting, back to that tick tock, tick tock scenario. Yehh there's my name. It's my turn. I must add that I had been waiting over an hour and a half, for a blood appointment that would take less than 5 minutes. Never mind, as it wasn't as if I was doing anything else.

Into the blood room I went, and would you believe it, Aidee my mate from Tameside works in that unit during the week. Brilliant. Familiarity. We had a chat whilst he took the blood and he told me that hopefully I would see him back at the Unit when I went for my last cycle.

Even though I felt ok, every time I had my bloods done, I feared that there would be something wrong. That one of the counts would not be as it should be and that it would interfere with my treatment plan, extending it even further. Thankfully, mine were always fine. They would only get in touch with you if there was a problem. No contact meant that it was full steam ahead for your next cycle.

The next day dawned and it was back down that M60. Same routine, mask and thermometer gun. I purchased a brew and some supplies at M&S because I had no idea how long I would be this time, so it was a butty and bag of crisps as well. No issues with my appetite.

It was the same long wait but eventually I was called up to the chemo suite. It was more scary, more clinical than at Tameside. So many more treatment chairs. So many people. There were lots of side rooms with about 10 chairs in each, but I was in a cubicle on my own. I could see patients in front of me, but not near enough to have any kind of chat. My cubicle was in 'pitstop 1'. I was pleased about this as I was right in front of the nurse's station.

This cycle was the change of drug I have previously mentioned, that potentially could give me an allergic reaction. I remembered what had happened to Sarah and can't lie, I felt really anxious. This time it was more like the images I had previously had in my mind of patients being given their chemo. There were so many people, lots of them looking really sad and poorly. I know it is selfish, but I did not want to see these things.

My cannula was put into my hand and the chemo syringe attached. The nurse was not required to sit with me this time so I was literally on my own. At least I could see the nurses. She told me that if I felt ill at any time, if I started with any kind of rash or my breathing felt tight, I must press my bell. I must have felt alright, as I ate my butty and crisps. I did convince myself at one point that my hands were coming out in a rash, but when the nurse looked she said that I was absolutely fine.

This cycle took just over an hour and thankfully went to plan. I was given my usual bag of drugs and syringes for the next 7 days and was told to keep an eye on my temperature and if there were any problems to ring the 24 hr Hotline. We had bought one of those gun type thermometers as believe it or not, we had never had one before.

Mr H was waiting over at the Maggies Centre – if you have never encountered a Maggies, please look them up. Another wonderful charity and in Greater Manchester we are so lucky that we have 2. I walked over to meet him, had a brew there and we were then on our way home so see what this drug might bring. Every time you have a cycle of chemo, it builds up cumulatively in your body, so potentially when you think that you may get used to it, the symptoms get worse due to the build up.

I would say that this cycle was similar to the first three in that nothing much happened, but actually, it was the worst one. Not that I was poorly or anything, but as you will read in a minute, it was the most eventful.

Strap yourself in for the events of the next few weeks.

Taken from my Facebook Post 19 July 2021

Good afternoon, on this wonderful, sunny if not a tad hot day.

Not checked in with you for a while so have a breather from what you are doing and we can have a catch up.

I have now had my 4th chemo which went without a hiccup and was quite uneventful. Back when I was told that I had to have the 6 rounds on 3 week intervals, those weeks/months seemed like a race with the ending so far away it was daunting. From that first one on the 7 May to the 5th one next week, well how quickly has that gone.

I have learnt now not to pack like I am going on a Sahara Trek, but it is hard when I usually take everything but the kitchen sink with me wherever I go. I mean, why wouldn't you! Don't tell me that it is just me, as I know some of you would be just the same.

Which brings me to my little 'Mini Break' at the 'Hotel Christie'. I know, I know, holidays are something that people have been desperate to do in these trying times and hopefully, you will be able to enjoy some leisure and holiday time quite soon.

Well, I managed to slip a quick 2 days in even before Boris said I could. What!! I hear you say.

To cut a long story short, and for the record, I am fine, I checked into the 5* Christie late one night. I had been having the usual 7 days of injections but this time, I was trying to get ahead of the game and prepare for day 7, to try and ward off the pains and back spasms. Mr H and I decided that we needed to speak with the 24 hour Hotline, just to check if I could start taking some strong painkillers a few days before. I thought it best to check, as you don't know if there are any contra-indications that would react with the chemo.

It was late in the evening when we phoned. They must have some kind of checklist of questions to ask when you phone them, the first one of which they asked being what my temperature was? I didn't know as it had been a few hours since I had taken it last and it had been fine, within the parameters we had been given. Thermometer gun in hand, Mr H fired it at my head. OMG 38.6 – yikes. But I didn't feel hot. How could it be that high.

Mrs Hotline was not happy with this reading and said we needed to try it again with a thermometer that you stuck under your tongue. Yikes, we didn't have one of them. It was like supermarket sweep. She said she would give us an hour to get one and then would ring us back, but in the meantime, she would need to speak to the on-call Registrar, as it was probable that I would have to go into hospital due to this temperature spike.

Mr H whipped down to Tesco and thankfully, they had a few in stock. We were still waiting for Mrs Hotline to phone so did the temperature check right away. In it went under the tongue and this, my friends is the only time in the whole of the chemo treatments that I was sick. I don't know if I was worked up about the prospect of going into hospital or what. But sick I was.

We waited and waited for that phone call. Mr H was not happy at the prospect of me having to go into hospital. I know that I had been in and out of various establishments since February, but actually being in hospital. Not happy at all.

Mrs Hotline phoned. We told her the reduced temperature but she was having none of it. The Registrar said he wanted me in and she was now going to book me a bed. I was to pack a bag and she would phone back to tell me when to come in.

I was catapulted into a right frenzy. I had no option - I had to go in. Help. By this time, it had gone midnight. I had had no preparation - what does one pack for such a stay? LV luggage OBVS, PJs, but alas in the rush to get sorted, when I got there, the bottoms did not match the top.

Going off on a tangent again. My friend Lesley who was a nurse, used to say to my Goddaughter, Emily, that if her knickers did not match her bra and she had an accident, the ambulance staff would not take her to hospital. Always sticks with me that ☺

For heaven's sake, my standards are slipping. What if I see someone I know, which believe me could be highly likely. I chucked in some underwear but the bigger dilemma was which 'hair' should I wear? Which bits of makeup will I need? I know, it's hospital I am going, not a fashion show but hey, that is just me. That's how I roll. I am who I am and it is too late to change now.

> Going on a trip.
> Need about 4
> outfits. I've packed
> 35 just to be safe.

Mr H is not happy about the prospect of me having to go into hospital. What about the VID! My temperature has come down slightly and he pleads with them not to admit me, but no. They want me in and I suppose it was better to be safe than sorry.
We arrive at the main entrance with said LV luggage. It is bizarre. There was not a soul about. No coffee at the M&S on the way past tonight.

Mr H had to hand me over to a very nice Security/Porter, who actually became more like my personal butler, fetching and carrying over the next two days, including 2 M & S deliveries from Mr H. Put it this way, he did not need to ask whom the stuff was for or where I was. He just knew. Now that was service.

2 trips to the M&S in Cheadle for Mr H with one Facetime - new PJs/shorts were purchased as it was so hot. Phew, normal service resumed – everything matches.

On admission, I was allocated a lovely male nurse who conducted every test under the sun. COVID obviously, MRSA, heart scan, water tested and much more. I was dripped up immediately to intravenous antibiotics. Very thorough but now I was, you guessed it, hungry. White toast and butter it was to be then. Yummy.

During that stay, I was treated to a ploughman's

lunch, right up my street, as I love a bit of cheese, in fact, it is my drug of choice. A full roast beef dinner that went down very nicely and of course the hospital breakfasts, white toast and butter once again, with a bit of marmalade thrown in for good measure.

I genuinely thought that I would be out the next day as surely there was nothing wrong with me. I felt fine. It was a long first day, but thankfully, I was in a room of my own so had full control of the TV and had taken plenty of reading material with me. When the Consultant eventually tipped up, she said that I had indeed got a slight infection, and I was going to have to stay in another day. Damn!! I suppose they know what they are doing though so stay I must.

I had to move rooms after the first night as the one I was in was just for Acute Admissions. Anyone who knows my holidaying from years gone by, know that I rarely stay in the first room I am given. On this occasion, I had to put a request in for said move not to be instigated until after 2200 hrs so I could watch 'Love Island' I know. I am trash TV junkie. Don't judge me. Permission granted. Can't knock a tryer.

New room, still my own but not quite as good as the first one. Yikes, no television, but luckily I have my iPad with me so all is not lost. This is not usually how it goes when you move rooms in a hotel, well not for me, I usually move to something bigger and better!

Alas not on this occasion though I am not complaining. This one was a bit like when you are put next to the building site. Well, let me tell you, there was a building site and by the end of my stay, the guy working with the deafening industrial staple machine was in great danger of having his ladder kicked from under him.

I digress, the upshot of this 'Mini Break' as I like to call it, though in fairness poor Mr H probably had more of a break not having to look after me, was that they concluded that I had an infection, that minor, they did not actually know where it was. So instead of a nice Aperol Spritz or Pink Prosecco, I was dripped up to fluids and intravenous antibiotics.

The good thing in all of this is that I did not feel ill or poorly, so that was a blessing. I probably looked the healthiest person in there.

So in good 'Trip Advisor' fashion:

- Accommodation – 5* tiptop. Own room, no single person supplement
- Food – 5*. Thumbs up to white toast and real butter, though not sure of the health benefits there but it was very nice. Roast beef and Yorkshire pudding too and not even a Sunday. Macaroni Cheese and a very nice rice pudding
- Entertainment – 5* 100% control of the remote

- Room Service – 5* Cannot fault my Private Butler
- Care and Compassion – 5* The staff were all wonderful, there are just too many patients and not enough nurses

Would I stay there again? Hell no, not by choice, but we are so lucky in Manchester to have this World Famous facility on our doorstep.

As far as 'Mini Breaks' go, I didn't find the Spa or the beauty salon, so always check the small print when booking.

Anyway, all that matters is that this was a small blip in my (cover your ears) it's the journey word again. I am safe, fit and well and that is what counts.

Much Love
Mrs H xx

Chemo 5 – Fifth Cycle – 30 July 2021

I am over my little holiday and now ready for cycle 5. 2 left. Almost there. It is the same procedure as last time. Bloods one day, chemo the next. No Aidee on blood day but yehh I am sitting waiting to be called for the chemo when there he was in front of me like my Guardian Angel. He checked how I was and I told him that I had been waiting ages. He disappeared upstairs and hey presto, there was my name on that big screen. Coincidence – maybe! When I went up, he came with me to my chair and sat with me for a while. It was little things like this that meant so much to me. People being kind. It's only a little thing but made such a difference.

If you can be anything in life, be nice.

The chemo again was straightforward. I count myself lucky that I did not have any adverse reaction and sailed through. This time though, I had started having an issue with my feet and my fingers. I now know this was Chemo Induced Peripheral Neuropathy (PN), and is why the nurses had started asking me how my feet were.

The chemo affects the sensory nerve fibres. It leaves you with sensations such as numbness, balance problems and pain. Some patients experience weakness of the muscles in the feet and hands. Some people do not get this and some get it far worse than I did. It is the luck of the draw.

Unfortunately, I suffered for many months with PN and at times thought that it would never go. It was tiresome to say the least as it was constantly there. It is one of the things that really got me down. I just wanted it to ease slightly to give me a break.

It is the strangest feeling and very hard to describe, but I will try. Imagine going out on a freezing cold night. You have your big thick socks on and warm cosy boots. Your feet however still get cold. You come home and off come the boots, your feet gradually warming up and you get those fuzzy sensations when you feel them coming back to normal. Not with PN. My feet felt warm to the touch but the messages going to my brain were telling me that they were not just cold, but painfully freezing.

This feeling was a constant throughout the day, but worsened as the night went on. I would sit with a smaller version of an electric blanket just trying to feel warm. As the months went on, these feelings gradually eased, with the feeling creeping back into them.

With the PN, your feet and sometimes fingers, feel as if you have just come in from the cold, but the feeling does not come back and the pain is awful. It is constantly there, in your every waking moment. They felt constantly numb.

I had it in both feet and in my thumbs and forefingers. I could not bear to wear any shoes or boots that enclosed my feet as it was just too painful and I felt like they were in a vice. Luckily it was Summer and I could live in flip flops.

Now I have many friends with lots of different skills but how lucky was I that I had Maria who is a qualified reflexologist. Bad news is that she lives 92 miles away, which makes it an almost 200 mile round journey and at least 2 hours each way. But make that journey she did, a number of times to work her magic on my tootsies. I lay back on my sun lounger whilst she administered her potions and worked away. It was glorious and relaxing and I cannot thank her enough. Just a pity she is so far away as I would be asking her to perform her miracles at every opportunity.

Shoes are one of my passions. I just love them. From being a little girl, I would get a new pair and immediately have to go outside to hear how they 'clicked' on the pavement. I would sneak into my mum's wardrobe and seek out the ones with the highest heels. I just love them.

High ones, sparkly ones, animal print, jewelled – you name them, I don't just like them, I love them. I cannot even hazard a guess of how many pairs I have. They are like my best friends, lovingly displayed in my dressing room – posh eh ☺

You can imagine then how I felt when I couldn't even get the lowest of shoes on. Like I said, flip flops, yes, and thankfully I have one or two pairs of them too. I felt like Cinderella desperately trying to force her toes into the glass slipper but feeling like the Ugly Sister as nothing fitted no matter how hard I tried.

I don't really possess what you would call – no, I

can't even bring myself to say the word!!! I will spell it out to you and you can say it out loud – curly c, umfy shoes. No, still can't say it. But to my horror, I had to admit defeat and go to that shop were you go when you are little to have your feet measured. See, I can't even say the name of the shop as it has connotations of – curly c, umfiness, and Velcro.

I am sure that you have guessed by now where I went then to get some of these shoes. I was not happy. Having said that, they do seem to have upped their game and have gotten more with it these days. However, if I see people of a certain age (I know ageist) buying there, it just puts me off. On this occasion, I had to bite the bullet and just get on with it.

I ended up with two pairs. Both were leather and with a kind of a metallic/goldish finish. The first pair a flat ballet type shoe and the second a trainer like shoe. To be honest, they are actually quite nice. Flippin expensive though. I draw the line at calling them the 'C' word ☺

I also bought a pair of Ugg slippers and the fur inside felt nice and soothing on my feet. This Neuropathy was proving to be costly to say the least. I must just add there that we were once in that particular shop and when checking out the price of something or other, Mr H commented that he thought they had missed an 'M' off the front of their name. Whoops ☺

I had to face the facts, that my precious shoes would not be going anywhere soon. I promised them that I would be back as soon as I could.

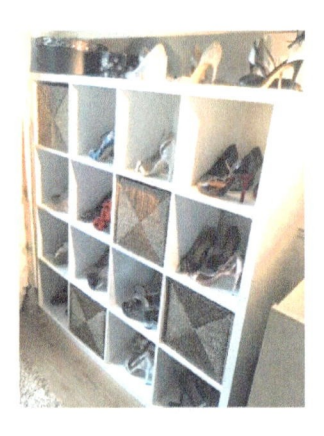

Another thing that plagued me after this cycle, and something they had warned me about, was the loss of nails. I have always, for as long as I can remember, taken care of my nails and worn varnish. Just the thought of them falling off made me feel sick.

Caroline, one the 'Oracles' had told me to try and keep them as short as I could. My fingernails funnily enough are quite long even when they are short. I have taken a hair, skin and nail supplement for years, so I hoped and prayed that this would pay dividend and that I would not lose any.

I had started to have regular pedicures which as well as being relaxing, also helped slightly with the PN, especially the massage. It was at one of these appointments that the therapist told me that two of my toenails were lifting. Oh SHIT – not actually said this for a while, but on this occasion it is definitely required.

They held on for a few days and then basically, dropped off during the night. Nice. There was however, a new nail already growing underneath, so not all was lost. The other ones were looking decidedly awful too. They were actually ghastly, particularly my big toes that looked like something heavy had been dropped on them. They were also riddled with what looked like some gruesome fungal infection. They weren't by the way.

The next visit revealed that another one was lifting. This was getting bad, but surely, I should now be getting a reduction in price, as I only had 7 nails to deal with ☺

There is something about nails don't you think? They are all well and good whilst they are happily attached to your body, but as soon as they leave, either by being cut or falling off, they turn into some vile, grisly, sickening body part. Like they have turned radioactive.

Tangent time – not had one of these for a while ☺ I was once on holiday, a quick week away in Tunisia. One of those weeks when you just wanted to fly and flop, relax and while away the hours. Alas, it was not to be. The Hotel left a lot to be desired, which is not like us as we are usually spot on with our choices. Well this one let me tell you, definitely left a lot to be desired!

There were many things that would make you cringe, but the final straw came whilst we were at the welcome meeting and staring straight at me, not attached to a human I may add, was a huge, yellowing toenail. One that looked like it had been clipped from a pre-historic animal. Do you remember when I told you that we rarely stay in the first room we are given on holiday? We went one-step further here, and actually moved hotels and now I think about it, resorts as well. I kid you not.

How ironic that the Hotel they sent us to, was one that we had visited almost 8 years previous. And this you won't believe, but it is absolutely true, the doorman said hello to us on the way in and said to Mr H "you've grown a beard since last time you were here"!

I realise that most of what I call the 'bad' things that happened to me were actually quite superficial. I am thankful and count myself lucky every day, as I know people who have had an absolutely stinker of a time whilst having their chemo. I am not trivialising it in any way and my heart and love goes out to anyone who has or is having a hard time.

To give hope to anyone who is suffering in this way, I am now 9 months on since my last chemo. My PN is almost under control and I would say from being 100% is now down to around the 10% mark. I know it is there, but it is manageable. Towards the end of the day, I get some pain and that freezing cold feeling, but I can deal with it.

You will be pleased to hear that some of my shoes have actually made an outing, though I still can't wear them for any length of time. I will get there though.

Chemo 5, in the bag. One more to go.

CHAPTER 17
CHEMO '6'
THE LAST ONE

Chemo 6 – Sixth Cycle – 20 August 2021

Don't be afraid to be your fabulous self, nobody will go blind if you shine too brightly
But rather, your light gives others silent permission to shine too

It is finally here, the last day of my chemo treatment. I can hardly believe it. At the beginning, I could not see the light at the end of the tunnel, but it is shining brightly, encouraging me towards it.

The only sad thing on that day was that the nurse that had looked after me the most, Thea, and the Health Care Assistant, Aidee, were not on duty. All the other staff were equally good but it would have been so nice for them to be there with me on that day.

I had made them both a 'goody bag' like the one that they gave me, but had things in that I thought they would like. Things to make their days easier. Thank you cards were bought, and words carefully written to express my thanks for everything they had done for me.

The chemo went as all the others, without any problem. How lucky had I been? The whole experience had not been half as bad as I had envisaged.

I absolutely feel for anyone that finds themselves in the same situation as myself, or in the need of any treatment for any other kind of cancer. It is SHIT and yes, I have said it again. But, we must have hope that with continued funding and research things will get even better than they are now. Early detection is also paramount in the success of cure and I will reiterate for the last time that if you are in any doubt about anything, you must go and see someone and get yourself checked out.

Ringing the Bell

Ringing the bell signifies the end of your treatment. I rang mine at the end of the Chemo. It was emotional for sure and thankfully, they let Mr H in for the occasion – he had gone through the mill as well.

There were a few blips along the way, but actually, it wasn't as bad as I expected. To a certain degree, I feel like I powered through chemo. I was lucky.

And you have guessed, correctly, the burning question that day was 'What to Wear'. Does my nail varnish match? Which shoes should I wear? And then, the unthinkable happened. As I was getting ready and just about to put my 'borrowed hair' on, I knocked the stand over and the 'Jeremy Jigg' (wig) fell into a cup of tea. Jeez, I had to squeeze it dry and hope the curls would re-form. My friend's husband told me that I had tea leaves in it later that day and I actually looked.

RING THE BELL

Ring this bell
Three times well
It's toll to clearly say
My treatment's done
This course is run
And, I am on my way
(J J Pennington)

CHAPTER 18
RADIOTHERAPY

September 2021

Radiotherapy is a treatment that uses high-energy beams of radiation focusing on cancerous tissue. This kills cancer cells, or stops cancer cells from multiplying. It is used mainly in addition to surgery.

5 treatments on consecutive days, though I had a weekend in between. I thought I would try my luck and see if I could go to the Macmillan Unit at Oldham Royal, which though about the same distance to 'The Mother Ship', is in a different direction, and even better has it's own car park. Permission granted. Yehh result.

Here is a Hindsy Tip if you wish to listen to me – never be afraid to ask a question, even if you think it's a cheeky or a daft one☺

The first appointment was to be measured and tattooed up. Tattooed, I hear you ask! Ohh a lovely butterfly or dainty flower. No such luck. Basically, a 'dot', well 2 'dots' that would mark the spot. Now these dots could easily be mistaken for freckles, of which I have many. Yikes, they could easily get lost trying to join the dots on my body.

I was taken into one of the radiotherapy rooms with equipment that looked like it belonged on the Star Ship Enterprise. I had been told that the actual radiotherapy was not at all painful so I was not scared, but just seeing the equipment sent a slight air of panic through my veins.

The technician explained what would happen during the actual treatment and that firstly she would need to do the measurements to ensure the radiotherapy would attack exactly the right spot. As mine was on the right hand side of my body, there would not be any issues around the heart area, which was good to hear.

She then brought in another technician, one to do the manhandling (not sure if I can say that in this world of political correctness, but hey, I have). It was however, a male of the species so I was actually correct in my description. It was bad enough having to reveal said boob in the first place, but having to do so to someone who looked like he had just turned up on his first YTS day, well, what can I say. That comment is probably 'ageist' too!! It's chemo brain. It makes you say the most strange, inappropriate things. Honest ☺

Before I hopped onto the bed, but not a bed in the

sense as it was all comfortable and cosy, I was given my 'Radiotherapy Gown'. This was to be mine for the duration of the treatment. A lovely navy blue number with Velcro fastenings for ease of access. Don't get me wrong, I love my labels, Ralph Lauren, YSL and the like but this one was firmly stamped up in all its glory with 'Oldham General Hospital'.

The bed, which actually was a hard bench like machine that moved in all directions, was my next port of call. I laid back and had to put my arms in stirrups behind my head. The technicians alternated between their computer screen, checking the measurements and manoeuvring my boob. Lifting it this way and that. You would think that by this stage I would be getting used to this kind of attention. But for me, not so. I hated it. But as they say, 'it is what it is' or 'it was what it was'. I just had to grin and bear it, if you pardon the pun.

When I was in the exact position, they marked me up. It was actually little more than a marker pen in reality and as I mentioned earlier, it just blends in with the rest of my freckles. However, these two were the most important ones I possessed, as they would be the guides to make sure that the treatment was going to the right place.

All done, appointments made. So far so good. Not painful at all.

My treatments were to be Wednesday, Thursday Friday and then the following Monday and Tuesday. Mr H took me to my first appointment, but they were still not allowing anyone else into the building with me, so once again I had to go it alone. There is a Maggies Centre on the Oldham Royal Hospital site so once he had said goodbye and parked up, that is where he headed for a brew and a biscuit.

I am sure that everyone's experiences of having 'Radiotherapy' are different, but for me, the experience was quite non-descript. After changing into the fetching blue number, I was called into the treatment room. Even more space like than the first one that I had been in, but actually had a very calm feel to it. The same torture like bed, but with another machine at the side, that I now know was the one that moved around me dishing out its 'rays'.

The first treatment took the longest, about 40 minutes, as they just could not get me in the right position. I was tipped backwards and forwards, up and down. My boob was lifted left, right and centre, plopped this way and that. It makes you feel like you are a piece of meat. The staff were all lovely and tried to put me at ease. To them, this was something they do every day but to me it was invasive.

Like most procedures, they tell you to 'relax'. How can you relax when you are basically half-naked, arms behind your back and two people who are alien to you are touching you up and down. I make this sound like something out of '50 Shades of Grey'. I felt like shouting a safe word but I do not think it would have worked in this situation.

I drove myself to the rest of the appointments, as I was familiar with the way there and knew there would be no issues with the parking. Treatment No 2, was slightly quicker than the first one and by No 3, I think they had sussed it. I was only actually on the bench for about 15 minutes, however, you have to keep as still as you can. I am prone to sneezing fits, hiccups and twitchy legs, but basically, I tried to not even breathe heavily for fear of my chest rising up and down too much. The technicians leave the room and watch you from a viewing gallery whilst the machine hovers over and around you, doing it's thing. It's a weird treatment, or at least mine was. You cannot see it and you cannot feel it.

The day of the final treatment arrived. I remember it being beautifully hot and sunny. I called into the supermarket on the way and bought a bag load of goodies for the staff. Donuts, pastries, cookies. All good stuff, that if I even look at, I put a lb on ☺

No 5 – boosh, done, finished. I handed back my 'designer' gown and thanked all the staff for their kindness.

That as they say, was that – finito – all treatment

finished. You would think that at this point I would have been elated. I walked out of that Macmillan Unit, walked to my car, got in and broke my heart crying. I think the enormity of what I had been through actually hit me. I should have been jumping for joy that it was all over but I felt scared, alone. For more than 12 months, I had had the most wonderful professional people looking after me. If I had a problem, they were there. If I needed anything, they were there. What was I going to do now? I felt as if I was being abandoned. It sounds silly. But the feeling for me was real.

Of course, I was not being abandoned. If I had any worries, these same people would still be at the end of the phone, ready and able to help me. Thankfully these feelings were short lived.

As I many have already mentioned, I don't really bare my soul to anyone. I am quite a closed book with my feelings. It maybe because I was an only child and did not have any siblings to share my thoughts or worries with. But actually, when I think about it, I did not really have anything to worry about growing up. I had a perfect life, with parents and family who loved me and cared for me. My formative life was actually trouble free. It is hard, therefore, to share my innermost thoughts and feelings.

There are things therefore, that whilst you read this book I am quite pleased that I have been able to share with you. My bestest of friends (of which there are many) will tell you 'I tell em nowt'! or the bare minimum that I feel they need to know. The only person that I confide in, is Mr H and that is good enough for me. It is not that I am secretive; it is just that I am immensely private.

CHAPTER 19
MOVING ON

It is now nearly October 21. How this year has flown. Nothing much to report really as the Pandemic is still raging and we are still required to isolate.

At least we have Christmas to look forward to. I do so love Christmas. I love the whole thing. I don't even mind the shopping or the wrapping up of the presents. It takes me an age though as I am finicky with the wrapping and everything has to match. Not for me the giving of gift vouchers. Oh no. I like to think about what people might like and hopefully, I get it right. I have never been told otherwise so will continue.

December looms. We are still in lockdown but Christmas is about to arrive at Hindsy Towers. Mr H builds the tree, which whilst it is not real, is very lifelike. Can't have any of those pesky needles hanging around for the puddies to eat. It is about 8 ft tall and very wide. It is his job to build and then put the lights on. That is where his involvement finishes.

Over the almost 24 years that we have been married,

I have collected many beautiful baubles. Nothing matches, but it all matches if you know what I mean. No red or green and definitely no tinsel. You will probably laugh at this and Mr H despairs, but I have to have my favourite two Christmas Albums on whilst decorating. The first one is not too bad and is Mary J Blige, Mary Christmas – so far so good. This is when it goes rogue. The second one is The Partridge Family Christmas Album. Who remembers the Partridge Family? David Cassidy☺ Don't knock it till you've tried it. It's a classic for sure.

Christmas Day 2021 is going to be good. Boris has said that we can have small gatherings this year (I will refrain from using the word 'party' - I could enlarge on that statement and get political in light of recent events – May 22, as that is where we are at the time of me writing this particular paragraph, but obviously, I won't). Our friends Pat and Dave are coming all the way from 'the rough end of the estate' (only joking, it's not that bad) and Chris's Mum, Mrs H Snr is coming from deepest darkest Cheshire. We will have an abundance of Real Cheshire Housewives that day.

As usual, I will be getting out my mum's best china, which though old is still actually very modern. The best cutlery (Mr H says that I have an obsession with cutlery sets, and this I cannot deny). The cutlery in question is a very nice Vilroy and Boch set, won by my Aunty Jose at one golf competition or other. She only let me have it on the proviso that it was used, so use it I do.

The preparations are going well. Everything is under control. Just under a week to go. I am just having a lazy morning and Mr H pops his head into the bedroom with a look of, well I don't know what on his face. He had been awake during the night with a bit of a tickly cough. He felt a bit odd. Well that wouldn't be anything new ☺ He had just done his lateral flow test (LFT) and was waiting for the result. Please NO. Oh shit – sorry for the bad language, again, but I think in this instance it is fully required – 2 lines as clear as day. It is the bloody VID! In true Victor Meldrew fashion, 'I don't believe it'.

In true Spandau Ballet style 'To cut a long story short', he had to go up to the local testing facility to have a PCR. When he came back, he suggested that I should do a test too. There was nothing wrong with me. Of that I was sure. So LFT for me it was. At least this was just an up the nose test, as you know what I am like with the down the throat test. I watch the test, willing it not to be positive. Does it really matter? If Mr H has it, I won't be going anywhere without him so we might as well both have it at the same time. One clear line, the other being that feint you could barely see it. Google however, advised that even the most feint line should be taken as a 'POSITIVE' result. Mr H had to make a second trip to the test centre with me. Now this was the dreaded

PCR. Oh no. Once again, it was not a pleasant experience. It just never got any easier for me and the 'singing' technique that I had previously used was not on this occasion successful. Say no more!!

We had to wait for the results that actually came back the next day – both positive, meaning that Christmas was once again - cancelled. A wash out. A disaster.

How strange that Positive, had been a word that had been just that during the previous year. It was an upbeat, encouraging, optimistic, confident, glass half-full word. Not on this occasion.

22 December 2021 Taken from my Facebook page

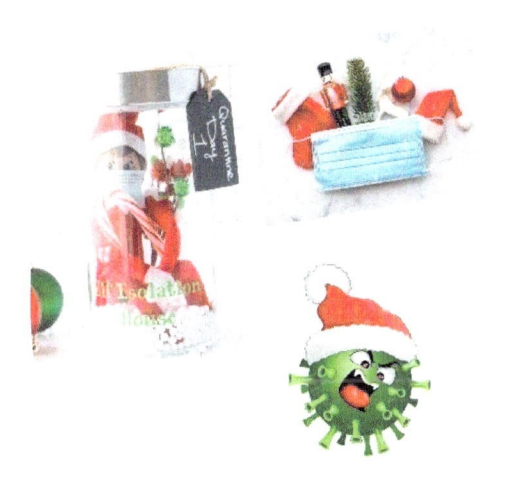

'Positive', unfortunately, is now well and truly

confirmed as the word of the day for Mr H & myself. Un-bloody-believable!!!

So that as they say is that - Christmas 2021 scuppered for us for this year. Cannot believe it and have no idea where we have both picked it up from. We have not been with anyone else who is positive. The only place that we have been together was M&S so if it was from there, it won't be just any old COVID. It will be an M&S COVID☺

Thankfully, we are both fully vaccinated and have had our boosters so hopefully, the way we are feeling will not get any worse. Strangely, after all my treatments this year, and everyone worrying about my vulnerability, Mr H is worse than me. I am obviously a tough cookie.

We had various things arranged for over the Festive Season, nothing wild or over the top and we were really looking forward to some normality after a tough year. Hey, ho, we will just have to have our planned Christmas in the New Year.

At least the isolation rules have lessened down to 7 days providing we have 2 negative tests on day 6 & 7.

So from Hindsy Quarantine Towers as it is now called, we wish everyone a safe and healthy Christmas and thank everyone who over the last year have been there for us both and got us through.

Also, my wonderful friends who have shopped once again for us, making sure that we don't run out of anything, though I did not realise that whiskey was classed as an essential!

On the plus side, we should be able to get a cheap turkey after Christmas.

31 December 2021 Taken from my Facebook page

Here is the Chris Whitty (Hinds) report, though actually, I am the witty one in our relationship☺

- Day 9 and Mrs H has 2 negative tests under her belt
- Mr H has 1 negative test, so here's hoping tomorrow is negative too

In any event, New Years Eve plans are cancelled, as 3 of our other friends who we should be celebrating with also have the VID and are in isolation.

My Christmas Tree, therefore, will be up for weeks the way we are going as we WILL be having our planned Christmas celebrations when we can.

Whatever you are up to, keep safe and respectful of others. Enjoy yourselves whatever you are up to and here's to a healthy and Happy New Year for us all.

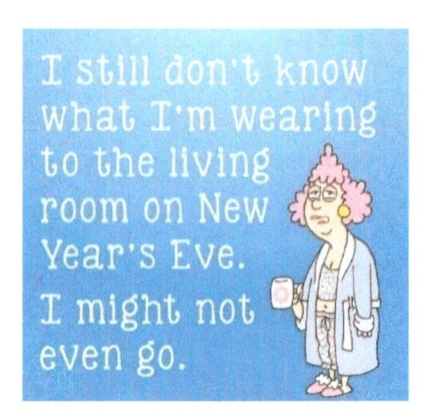

9 January 2022 Taken from my Facebook page

As you know, we did not have our planned Christmas due to the VID, so we are having it next week. Yehh The tree is still up and I can hear the superstitious ones amongst you gasping that it is 'bad luck'. Hey, it can't bring anything worse than last year so I am willing to take a chance. Up it stays.

Our Christmas Eve will be at Chez Massey (Pat & Dave's) with Helen & David and Mrs H Snr. We will have our Secret Santa, games, good food and company and on Christmas Day, it will be Christmas Day Dinner at ours, with all the trimmings.

We managed our isolation New Year's Eve meal as Romiley Golf Club kindly did a take out for us and the no-VID friends delivered it. We then had a 3 hour Zoom. Brilliant.

Merry Christmas and Happy New Year from Hindsy Towers and here's to a fabulous, healthy and prosperous 2022.

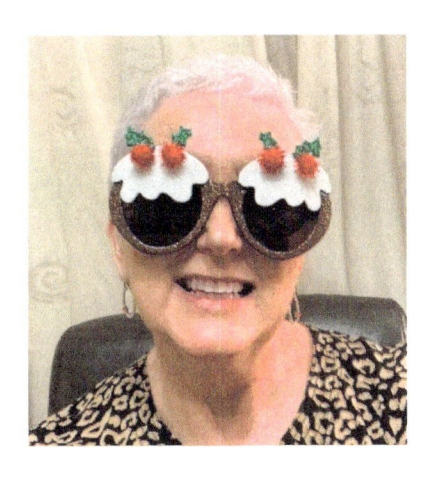

FEBRUARY 2022

4 February 2022 - *from my Facebook page – 4 February 2022 – feeling grateful*

4th February is World Cancer Day so it feels right to update you with what had been going on at Hindsy Towers.

Get a cuppa and strap yourself in for a little old read.

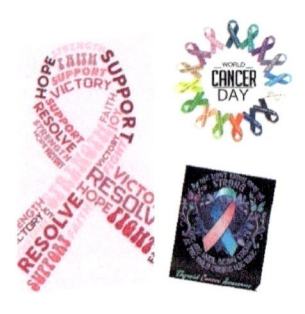

All is well at Hindsy Towers and almost back to some kind of normal, whatever that now looks like. I am now back on the 'Slimming World Waggon', as what with the pandemic, chemo and radiotherapy the lbs were not kind to me. Well they thought they were being kind, as they did not want to leave me. But thanks to my Slimming World Consultant, Rob and my friends at class, I have already said goodbye to almost 2 stone.

I had been wearing my wigs constantly throughout my treatment because as confident as people think I am, some things were just too hard. I literally take my hat off to those who go wigless. I only ever did this in the house with Mr H. Even my most trusted friends and family never saw me without it. People say it doesn't matter. You are you, it doesn't matter what you look like and that being well is what matters, but to me, it really did matter.

As I have previously told you, I had three different wigs, in various lengths and colours. I used to joke if I put weight on that it was most definitely because of my heavy wig, or if I lost weight, that it must be because I had shed another few toenails, or the hairs were growing on my legs! (that is most definitely a positive side effect).

Physically, my hair is doing really well and if you see me out and about, I will be sporting my inner 'Annie Lennox' look. All home grown now with flickering eye lashes, well not quite, but they are definitely coming back. And, I am now in possession of a full set of toenails

It was on my weekly visit to SW as I will now call it, that I pulled up in the car par, looked in the mirror to reverse and shrieked. OMG, I had forgot to put my wig on. Panic. I rang Mr H and said that it was his fault because he had let me go out of the house without it. He said that as he was used to seeing me without it, he really didn't notice. Bless, he said he would drive down with it, but by the time he would have got there the class would have been over.

I had two choices, either go home and run for the hills or, bite the bullet and go in. I quickly fluffed up what bit of hair I had, which in fairness, was looking like a really short elfin like cut and in I went.

In my head, the voices were telling me that everyone was looking. My heart was beating fast and I could feel tears in my eyes. I hadn't wanted this to happen. I wasn't ready. I had nothing to fear. Rob and the ladies at my class are absolute diamonds and couldn't have put my fears to rest any better. I was going to be ok. That was my turning point, I never wore the wig again.

My 'peripheral neuropathy' is now only a slight annoyance instead of being a constant drain on my senses. It was not without humour though as I managed to flip a whole bottle of nail glue all over my hand as I thought I had hold of the bottle but didn't. Result – a fully stuck hand, rings stuck to my skin and together and skin that looked like it was falling off. Awful at the time but funny now.

Plus, the occasional fall off the front step as I couldn't feel the floor. I still demand a foot rub every night as 'it is medical, don't you know'. Mr H swears that his fingerprints are wearing out and in this age of technology, heaven help us if he can't get into his mobile phone. I have sent him to The Priory once before for similar.

I have my first BREAMO – Breast Moving On – appointment later this month. First mammogram and discussion about the way forward. Understandably anxious but it is necessary and they will look after me well at the Nightingale. Can't say I am looking forward to the squishy, squashy machine again though. Women know exactly what I mean, but for men, imagine putting your 'you know what' in a photo copier and pressing on really hard – ouch.

MRS H'S STORM IN A D CUP

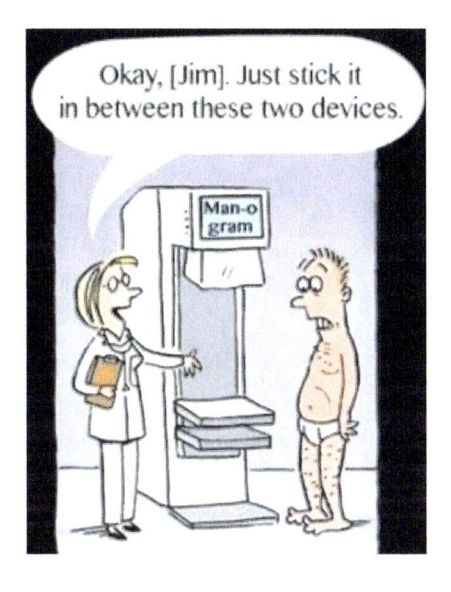

The point of this post is to remind you that it is World Cancer Day. I have at least 25 people in my circle of friends who specifically have had breast cancer and are all survivors. All amazingly strong. I have two friends who are at the end of their treatment and I wish them love, strength and support now to get them back to their new normal.

I have been on two courses, albeit on Zoom, with the Look Good Feel Better Charity. A course for skin and makeup and one for scalp and hair care. A brilliant Charity helping people to make the best of themselves. They offer many different types of course. Have a look online. You never know when you may know someone who it will help.

Likewise, the Maggies Centres are amazing places

and in our area, we are lucky we have two available to us. Mr H and my friends' husbands have used their facilities whilst waiting for us to have our treatment at The Christie. No questions asked as to why you are there or how long you will be. They just envelope you in love and kindness. Have a look what they have to offer.

So on this awareness day it is the usual message that I will keep reiterating, 'If in Doubt, Check it Out' – Remember, no question is a daft question.

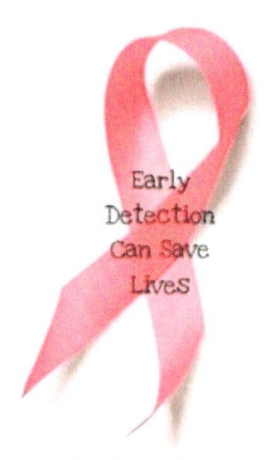

It is a scary place to be but the treatments and care we have available now are so much better than years ago and with continued research, it can only get better.

Much Love
Mrs H xx

THE MIRROR

I lift my eyes
I see me
A tear falls
The person in the mirror
She is different
Her skin pale, her eyes sad
She looks back at me
Her eyes of sorrow show the emotion
It's almost like she knows me
Remembers me
Wonders where I have been
Why do you look different? She asks
Without a word spoken
I had cancer
(Dana Stewart)

CHAPTER 20
APRIL/MAY 2022

I thought about writing this book way back in 2021. During the nights when I could not sleep for one reason or another. I lay there and ran through in my mind things that I would write. There was some good stuff. I even made myself laugh, and sometimes cry. I remember thinking I will write that down tomorrow, but I never did. I have had to dig deep to try to remember what I wanted to say. The 'journey' began - yes, I know, I've said it again. But what other word could I use? It could have been an expedition or a voyage. It has however, been a journey of epic proportion. A journey through my thoughts and feelings, hopefully some useful facts, an insight into my life over the last year and I hope I have brought some of my personality and humour too.

I have thrown myself back into fundraising, but I am now spreading the net further afield trying to help some smaller charities.

I firstly dipped my toe in by organised a small event for Mossley Cancer Committee, to ease myself back into raising money. With the help of my two wonderful friends, Darren and Chris of Mr Finch & Skin in Ashton - look them up, a fabulous haven of a shop with heavenly products but more than that, two guys who I love dearly and have been a constant support to me. We put on a small event in the salon for 7 of my friends who benefited from treatments from Chris. Darren & I kept everyone amused and we had a bit of a buffet and a couple of glasses of fizz. It would have been rude not to! £355 in the pot.

On one of my visits to the Cancer Warriors in Stalybridge, we got talking about wigs and alternative therapies and how important, particularly my wig was to me. They were looking at converting one of their rooms into a wig room so I said that I would do a charity event for them. The benefit of knowing lots of people, and believe me when I say, I know a lot of people, is that I usually know someone who can step up to the plate and help. My wonderful friend Natalie Bagley, from up at Bees Coffee Pot up on Harrop Edge – a bit like Alderley Edge but nicer - did just that. Another strong, caring lady. Easter weekend therefore was spent up at the Coffee Pot, raffle tickets at the ready along with a couple of stalls that Nat had arranged. The weather was good and it was a busy few days. I seconded my friend Alison to help and I think she is now my 'fundraising apprentice'. Obviously, Mr H was on duty too. We come as a double act. The Jo and Chris show (I've put this in as it always winds him up that everyone always says my name first and that alphabetically it should be him ☺). A fabulous effort by all and £1,062 in the pot.

Our biggest event since lockdown was a concert for Willow Wood, with music by Ashton-Under-Lyne Brass Band. It was the Friday before St George's Day so they played all the Last Night of the Proms favourites. We held it in the Albion Church in Ashton, a fabulous venue for the acoustics. Mr H applied for a drinks license. A gamble as we had not done this before but it definitely paid off. Flags were purchased, and lyrics to the songs projected onto a big screen. We had an army of helpers and in particular, the McClure family were invaluable along with Laura & Heath, although the latter drank his own body weight in beers whilst serving, but at lease he paid for them.

I am not usually a stress head, but because this was a 'big gig' and we had the outlay for all the booze, I was nervous. Mr H though, took everything in his stride. I should have took a leaf out of his book, as it was a massive success. Just to hear the band and see everyone stood waving their flags and singing their hearts out was uplifting itself. This is now going to be an annual event as the feedback was so good. £2,317 in the pot.

WELLBEING DAY

Wellbeing is a word that we hear more and more of these days. Companies looking after their employees and caring. How good would it be if people just cared that little bit more.

How lovely was it then when Sarah one of my 'oracles' invited me along to my previous place of work, you know the place where they chase baddies and lock them up,! They were having a 'Wellbeing Day' and Sarah had invited an Ambassador from the Prevent Breast Cancer Charity (another Sarah) to come along. It had been 3 years since I had left so felt quite strange driving down that road. It was great to see so many of my old colleagues.

Earlier in the day, Sarah and some of her team had been around the building wielding a false pair of boobies that contained multiple lumps. The idea was that staff would have a 'good feel' and it would be educational about how to check yourselves and also to reiterate the importance of making sure that you attend those mammogram appointments. In true GMP style, there were also boxes of donuts making the rounds, but these were in the shape of boobies, nipples and all. The idea was to raise awareness but also to raise money too. Which they did, lots. They got the guys involved too which was good as don't forget, breast cancer can affect men too.

It was a beautiful hot day and as part of the 'Wellbeing' they had two officers, the beefcake type, who were putting anyone who was brave enough through what I describe as a mini boot camp. Of course, if I would have known, I would have taken my gym kit with me – I think not ☺ and in any event, I had me gold heels on ☺They were put through their paces and from my bench, it looked like they were having a good, if not sweaty time. I did, however, don a pink tutu for the obligatory 'Instagram' photo with said beefcakes. I think having an 'Instagram' board is the way forward as it can hide a multitude of sins☺

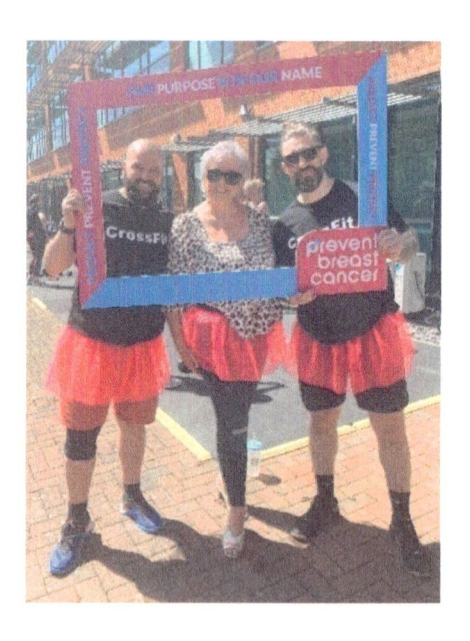

Well done Sarah xx

SLIMMING WORLD

I have mentioned numerous times the other road I constantly find myself driving down. Over the years, I have tried almost every diet going – Weight

Watchers, Rosemary Conley, Atkins and many others. I think where I failed was that I did them all on the same day ☺ SW is the only one that works for me, it may not work for others, but it does for me. Where I have fell down in the past is that once I have hit that target, I have become complacent and stopped going to class, thinking I knew best and that I could go it alone. Wrong. I need that accountability, the peer pressure and the standing on those scales, though sometimes I do not like them!

I have always been tall, though as I get older, others seem to be catching me up, but when I was young, I was always the one on the back row, always that tall girl. My dad's side of the family are all tall, strong specimens. When the weight started to creep on, people would say that it was because I was tall. I could carry it. Well that was right because carry it I did. I always said it was because I had heavy bones – who knows I might have but it's a bit hard to weigh them. I most definitely carry a considerable amount of weight in the chest department and that never seems to change. It may also be that I have a heavy brain, though I doubt it very much.

The SW class I attend is at East Cheshire Harriers, and believe me when I say that that is the nearest I will ever get to a running track! I thought, therefore, that I would enlighten you with some of the hilarious rituals that go on at our SW class, as well as supporting each other, the laughs we have along the way keep us going.

There are the mandatory rituals that we have to adhere to each week:-

- To start with there is the pre-weigh in tea. NIL by mouth after 7pm and if you do have to eat, most definitely the lightest meal you can find. Not much time you see to get rid of any extra lbs that may lie in wait
- Weigh day arrives and you have to make another good choice in what clothes to wear. They have to be lightest you can possibly find. In the depths of winter SW members can be found in their flimsy Summer dresses and flip flops. Always thinking
- Do NOT even think of wearing that padded bra with the wires – every ounce counts
- Even though you will have had your first tinkle of the day, you must always go when you get to class to try to squeeze out that last bit of excess liquid
- If you can get a 'No 2' in as well, that would be amazing. I have never yet been able to get my ablutions in line with weigh day – gross I know☺
- Under no circumstances must breakfast or a beverage of any kind be consumed before

class – beware therefore that you do not get crushed in the post weigh in rush to the coffee facilities or the SW biscuits

- If you do have to wear shoes or accessories of any kind, you must always remember to strip to the bear minimum before your feet touch those scales – that includes the removal of belts, watches, jewellery of any description and anything that may tip you over the edge
- Once you approach the scales, you need to step on in the most delicate way you can, so as not to shock them
- Lean forward and stick your bum out to try to get the balance of weigh just right. If needed and if you are able, lift those bosoms up too
- Not too much you can do about this one, but we have members that as soon as they hit the M60 on the way to the airport, balloon and bloat up, and this gets even worse once up in the air – we have decided as a group that being high up, definitely increases weight. I think then that my height and the fact that I live almost 900 feet above sea level most definitely is a factor for me!! East Cheshire Harriers is over 500 feet lower than Hindsy Towers. Could it be that I am not overweight and it is merely the gravitational pull of the earth making me weigh heavier☺
- Our beloved leader 'Rob' says that he lives

> near a reservoir and therefore his excuse is that he must have water retention☺

There are then those people who have hit their target – grrrr – and continue to lose weight and have to go home to 'eat cake'. They are the most hated people in group - (only joking – they are our inspiration).

You understand now why this losing weight lark is so difficult. There are dangers lurking in dark corners everywhere.

I had done really well prior to lockdown. I had said goodbye to 3 stone and was feeling good about myself. Clothes were fitting well and I was walking with that slight swagger you get when you are pleased with yourself.

Enter the VID stage left!!! Being at home did not do anyone any favours. Try as I did, it was just too hard to make good choices all the time. Remember those days when you literally had to buy what they had on the shelves.

My 'annus horribilis' didn't help either. Steroids were not kind to me, though it could have been a lot worse. We were treated to copious afternoon teas and many other delicacies, all of which were very gratefully received but alas, have stayed with me longer than I would have liked.

Going to group is now a part of my weekly routine. I will get to that target, come what may, though it may take me longer than I originally thought. I am lucky that the group I attend is full of wonderful people who are all supportive of each other, all chasing the same goal.

When I went back to group in October 21, it wasn't without trepidation and anxiety. I need not have worried. Everyone welcomed me back, with open arms, and I feel that they are part of my life. They were and are a great support to me and we encourage each other. It's not like a slimming club, fat club or whatever you want to call it. It is like going for a coffee with a group of friends, chatting over the weeks' events, sharing ideas and tips but not forgetting those 'blasted scales'.

I am going to the Prevent Breast Cancer ball soon and just need to lose a few extra pounds before I start deciding what to wear. I will be proud to attend that event and will wear my badge with pride.

THE NEW NORMAL

LIfe therefore Is almost back to normal. I had my BREAMO appointment, my first mammogram and thank god, it was clear. I am back at work, remember those 16 hrs that are easing me nearer to retirement. I have just had a birthday and it was lovely to be able to celebrate in the company of good friends. We have a few nice things to look forward to – Tears for Fears at an outdoor venue in Scarborough, supported by Alison Moyet. Afternoon Tea at the Midland Hotel in Morecambe. Jane Macdonald at the Lowry. South Pacific at the Palace Theatre Manchester and hopefully lots more. I am going away to Turkey with three of my Police family and then Mr H and I are going on our first cruise next year. We will be both hitting the big '60' and it is also our Silver Wedding. Much to celebrate.

I have just had my first 'big girl haircut' since my hair has come back. I wasn't expecting a cut, just a blow dry and that salon experience that I have so missed. Before I knew it, Gemma had her scissors to hand and was snipping away. I think I may have got used to it being short, so this may be the new me, or maybe not. Need now to make the decision as to what colour I am going to be or not, as I may stay with my new silver, grey locks. It is up to me, I can do whatever I want. When I lost my hair, I feared that it would not come back. I was scared that this was how it would be forever. We are never happy with what we have and always want something else. When you don't have curls you want them and when it is straight, you want curls. I have learnt to be grateful for what I have and will embrace it the best I can.

I am on 5 yearly mammograms, though I have already had one, but I think I will not be able to cope with that and will have them forever. I am on a tablet (Letrozole) for the next 10 years.

Letrozole is a medicine used for treating breast cancer. It can also help prevent breast cancer coming back. It is mainly prescribed for women who have been through the menopause and have a type of cancer called "hormone-dependent" breast cancer.

One good thing that I did not know, is that I have already gone through the menopause. Yeh, that's one less thing for me to worry about. Like all medications, there are side effects. Weight gain!! I think I will be dieting forever, but I will continue to try and keep to a healthy weight, as the benefits of taking the tablets outweigh not taking them. I am suffering with joint, bone and muscle pain, but I will muster on and plan to get back on my bike soon.

I am also going to start swimming. Don't be under any illusion though, an Olympian I am not. I am more of a don't get your hair wet kind of girl that just glides up and down. I have bought a new swimming costume and a new towel. All I need to do now is actually join the gym!!

Tangent Time

It would be rude of me not to add a little 'tangent' here, as by now you should be used to them.

I have just come back from a wonderful weekend in

JOANNE HINDS

Anglesey with my lovely friends Janet and Neil and their family. We basically barged in and joined them. We stayed in a quaint little Welsh B&B, exactly as you would imagine one to be. A farmhouse handed down through the generations with Mrs Roberts the perfect host. Rickety stair rails and creaky floorboards, all adding to the experience.

B&B breakfasts are always the best. Full English with all the trimmings and homemade marmalade and toast with lashings of butter. Copious pots of freshly brewed coffee adding to the amazing smells coming out of the kitchen.

Mrs Roberts, or Joyce as she was called was telling us that she was going to some friends that afternoon and had a chocolate cake in the oven. And here it comes, both of her friends have recently had breast cancer and they were having a get together to raise some money.

She was telling us that one of the ladies had written a book – oh yes, so it's not just me!! That chemo must get those creative juices flowing for sure. However, this book was about what this lady was going to do, and that was climb the three peaks. WTF!!! I can just about climb the stairs without my legs giving in on me. It must be that Welsh air.

In an effort therefore not to be outdone, I decided that I too would do '3' of something. You will be pleased to know, that there will be no mountains involved, or even smallish hills. I am going to do the '3 shopping centres' – the three peaks are just so last year. I will be starting with the Trafford Centre, then moving on to Cheshire Oaks (fresh air hit for that one) and finishing off with Meadowhall in Sheffield. That will get some steps in ☺

All in all, it was a year and a half to be sure, and one that I never want to re-live again. I think I must reiterate again how lucky I was. To be diagnosed in the first place, to have not missed any appointments, to have sailed through my chemo and radiotherapy as best I could. I did not have many emotional days but there were some crappy cancer days. I hope that anyone who is not quite strong enough or does not have a Mr H like me, can get the support they need as it really matters.

My body has been through a lot, but there was only ever one option, to keep going, keep smiling and keep laughing.

I am back in the game

ACKNOWLEDGEMENTS

Hello and thank you for sticking with me and reading about my 'Storm in a D Cup'. I hope you enjoyed it.

Once I got going, I really enjoyed writing this book and I would say, if you fancy doing something you have never tried before, give it a go. For me it was very therapeutic, though sometimes, emotive.

I didn't really know how much I would or could write. Mr H said that it should be somewhere near the 40,000 words mark for a standard paperback. OMG, I was never going to reach that in a month of Sundays. I told him that I wasn't even sure I knew that many words. His response was that I most certainly did, and he has to listen to them and more every day. Cheeky ☺ By the time I finish, I will be somewhere near the 44,000 word mark which I am actually amazed by. It is that bank training. Give me a target and I will always hit it and usually exceed it.

Fact/Myth – Do women talk more than men?

Apparently, men speak about 7,000 words a day and women about 20,000. I think the reason for this is that men don't listen properly, and women have to repeat themselves numerous times☺ Controversial I know, but by now you will know that I don't care☺

Mr H always knows when I have not had much contact with anyone as he says that I go into overdrive and definitely exceed my daily quota!

Unlike JK Rowling, I did not do my writing in a coffee shop in Edinburgh. Most of it was whilst I sat at the kitchen unit and sometimes on a cushion, propped up in bed. My trusted cats were never far from my side and indeed, Georgie would sometimes try to get in on the act, as he is most certainly a fan of trying to sit on the keyboard.

My cats were a constant source of comfort to me. Georgie in particular. He most definitely picked up on my anxieties and whereas he follows me round on a normal day, he stuck to me like glue. (jeez, I almost spelt definitely wrong – that could have been a whole new episode in Line of Duty – if you know, you know, and if you didn't watch it, you missed a trick).

Serendipity, the little Princess, though never too far away, wasn't really arsed. But Mr Bojangles, our BoBo, our beautiful Maine Coon though usually ensconced somewhere with Mr H, did his regular checks on me. We were heartbroken when suddenly on Valentines Day 2022, he had what we think was a heart attack whilst sat on Mr H's lap and passed away. We had been through so much and were just getting back on track and then this happened. We were devastated, and still are. We miss him immensely. Why is life so cruel?

My inspiration to write this book came from Mr H and a few of my friends who said they liked the way I wrote and gave me encouragement. I am almost at the end and feel immensely proud of myself. I cannot wait to see it in print. I may even have one of those book launches with a few glasses of prosecco thrown in, one of those pink balloon arches and some booby cakes.

As well as the question of what I wanted to achieve by writing the book, I was also asked about my budget. Another alien thing to me☺ Even if I had one, I would most definitely go over it. I don't think I will make my fortune, but I am not bothered. If it helps just one person, if it gives someone a giggle, if it raises awareness, it will have been worth it.

Mr H is a very special person who has always there for me, whatever. He is positivity in a can. He was there, when he was able to be (flippin pandemic) every step of the way and my health, wellbeing and happiness is what he wants for me in life. He has been on hand all the way through, listening to me tapping my way through this book and is probably glad it's finished and he doesn't have to hear 'just come and listen to this bit, does it sound ok?'.

Apparently, I hold my breath when I am typing, so he had to tell me to breath on many an occasion☺

Mr H

My Mr H. My dad told him before he died that he had to look after me. Little did he know to what extent and to what lengths he would have to travel to do so. He has gone far and beyond, looking after me like a precious stone and carried me safely along life's pathway, though sometimes it has been rocky and I have been like a wobbly jelly.

We have stormed through life's adventures together. Some funny, some crazy, some sad and some scary. Together, we get through the rough and the smooth. I have already told you, but in case you skim read that bit, it is our 25th Wedding Anniversary next year (2023) and we will both be 60. Apparently, I need to think of 25 amazing things that we can do together.

It is going to be one hell of a year.

His calmness to a situation is infectious; though sometimes I crack, he is always the calm in my storm.

> *He is my life and my love, not just today but every*
> *Day*
> *I love you – your Mrs H*
> *xxxxx*

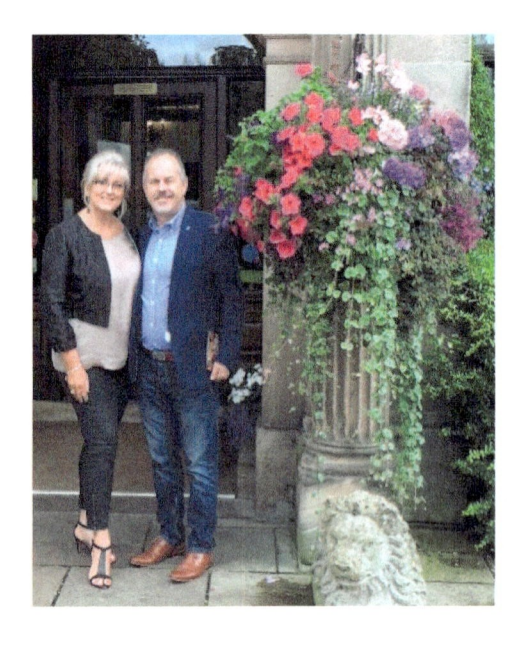

Not long after my diagnosis, I started to think about other people I knew who had also had breast cancer like me and were still here to tell the tale. They were all either in my immediate friends group or people I know through friends. The number astounded me – all wonderful brave ladies. So many of them.

Whilst I have been on my 'journey,' – oh no, I had to get another quick one in before the end, and for the record, I have just done a quick check, and there have been 13 journeys mentioned. 13 is not lucky so this one makes 14 so we are ok ☺ - there were 4 other friends going through exactly the same as me, though we all have different stories to tell.

I want therefore to dedicate this book not only to those beautiful, brave ladies, and wish them all health and happiness in everything they do, but also to anyone who has walked in the same shoes and are breast cancer survivors.

Aunty Jose (Hankinson) - Narraine Oldham
Christine Barry - Sarah Aldred
Joyce Vernon
Danielle Nutter - Dr Janet Rubener
Sheila Bellavia - Caroline Hall
Deborah Leach - Carol Dean
Nicky Lavery - Carol White
Marion Marsh – Pat Walklate
Ann Leach - Anne Drahme
Nicola Duerden - Karen Valentine
Trish Callan - Sarah Houghton
Jinette Lunt   Joanne Biggs
Nita Jhanjii-Garrod

I also want to thank the staff and volunteers who run the following Organisations who were paramount to both Mr H and myself, providing support, kindness and in some cases a good brew.

David Banks and his team and the Chemo Nurses from The Christie who work out of the Macmillan Unit, Tameside.
The Maggies Centres at Oldham and Manchester - I know that they have also been a great source of comfort and help to a few other people I know who have gone through or who are still going through various types of cancer.

Cancer Warriors, Stalybridge – a very small local charity who are similar to the Maggies in that their door is always open. You will be met with a smile and a welcome, and again, a right good brew.

Valerie Lee and her wonderful team of volunteers at Mossley Cancer Committee. Another local charity that has been going for over 50 years. They have an amazing band of supporters, raising money throughout the year and distributing it to deserving recipients throughout Tameside. Valerie is a force to be reckoned with and throws herself into not only MCC fundraising, but also many other community events and activities. She is a true angel.

Day Services, Reflexology Therapist at Willow Wood Hospice – I was lucky enough to be able to attend Willow Wood and benefit from the wonderful experience of reflexology. This was when my neuropathy was causing me pain and discomfort. It most certainly helped relieve some of the symptoms and it was just nice to be able to lie back for that hour in a relaxing, uncomplicated environment. I have been a volunteer there for over 13 years but never imagined that I would need any of their services. Mr H and myself are both back in full throttle with our fundraising for them so that with our help and the help of others, the future of the Hospice can be secured.

Prevent Breast Cancer – We first knew of this Organisation when we met up with Clare who is a volunteer at Maggies. Mr H offered his services to do them a free website for their 'Creative Writing Group' which was made up of cancer patients. As well as being a volunteer at Maggies, she is involved with PBC.

PBC has since 1996 been working hard to eradicate breast cancer for future generations. They have achieved great things. They are located at the Nightingale Centre and feed into the Prevention Programme at the Christie.

Their mantra is, Predict, Prevent, Protect. Powerful isn't it!

All proceeds for this book will be split between some wonderful charities that have been paramount to me.

- Cancer Warriors, Stalybridge
- Mossley Cancer Committee
- Prevent Breast Cancer
- Willow Wood Hospice

And of course, it would be rude of me not to mention all my family and friends who kept both Mr H and myself going with their love and support, flowers and food. I do not have many immediate family members, so my friends as they say are the family I chose. Aunty Jean and Carol, my Hospice Partners joke that I have a 'Top 10' and they sometimes sneak in there. In reality, I have many, many friends and love them all.

And lastly, I could not end my 'Storm in a D Cup' without mentioning with ultimate love, pride and affection, the two women in my life who sadly are no longer with me.

My mum, who sadly passed away when she was only 64 years old, after bravely and with so much dignity battled for many years. She was my everything, and she left a hole in my heart that will never heal. She never complained and was compassionate and caring to others right until the end. She, along with my dad only ever wanted the best for me and for me to be happy in life. She never got to meet Mr H, but I know she would have approved. I hope she knows that I am very happy.

The other lady is my wonderful Aunty Beryl, my mum's sister. Growing up, we were a tight knit family and we were just always together. She was love itself. She led a simple life and never asked for anything (well perhaps my dad to mend her iron, of which she went through many). She too fought to the end with dignity.

JOYCE MIDDLEHURST

BERYL HAND

JOANNE HINDS

Thank you for purchasing this book. I am pleased to tell you that 100% of every £10 book sold will be split equally between the following 4 charities that are close to my heart. I am delighted to say that all four charities will be getting at the least £400 which I am absolutely over the moon with and cannot thank you all for supporting me in this venture.

Much Love
Mrs H

Prevent Breast Cancer
Registered Charity No: 1109839

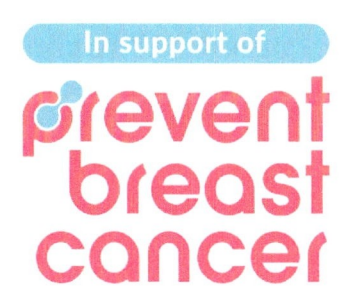

Prevent Breast Cancer is the only UK Charity entirely dedicated to the prediction and prevention of breast cancer, committed to freeing the world from the disease altogether. Unlike many cancer charities, we are focused on preventing, rather than curing. By promoting early diagnosis, screening and lifestyle changes, we believe we can stop the problem before it starts. And being situated at the only Prevent Breast Cancer Centre in the UK, we are right at the front-line in the fight against this disease.

Tameside & Glossop Hospice (Willow Wood)
Registered Charity No: 1029318

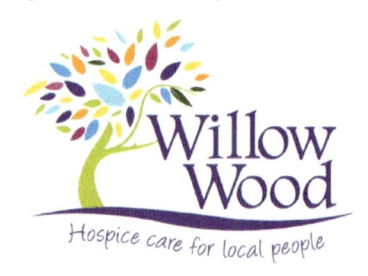

Willow Wood Hospice provides adult specialist palliative care for patients with life limiting illnesses, both cancer and non-cancer diagnosis. They provide care, free of charge and patients' families and their carers are at the centre of everything they do.

They aim to help everyone who passes through the doors to attain the best possible quality of life. Care whether it be physical, psychological, social or spiritual also extends to families and partners. they offer a number of services including an In-Patient Unit, Day Services Unit, Dementia support and Bereavement Counselling.

Mossley Cancer Committee

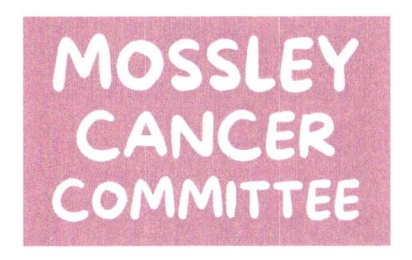

Mossley Cancer Committee supports cancer charities locally in the Greater Manchester Area. The committee distributes funds to support any person afflicted by cancer and related diseases, including the provision of comforts, medical aid and any other matters connected with the alleviation of suffering or the amelioration of their life, and also, to encourage the research into the cure of cancer and the said associated diseases and the cause thereof

JOANNE HINDS

Cancer Warriors (Stalybridge)
Registered Charity No: 165851

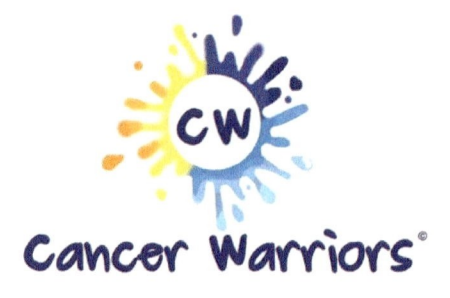

Locally, nationally and internationally, Cancer Warriors is a vocal advocate service for cancer awareness and support. Our core value is to make sure that no one has to deal with cancer alone.

With over 10 years' experience (Est 2007, Cancer Warriors has devoted its energy to passionately advocating cancer for the local community, whilst raising funds for The Christie NHS Trust & Macmillan Cancer Support.